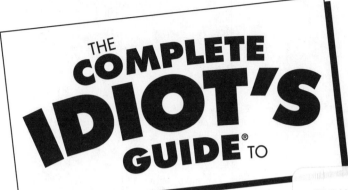

THE
COMPLETE
IDIOT'S
GUIDE® TO

D0564948

Healthy
Weight Loss

Second Edition

Lucy Beale,
Sandy G. Couvillon, M.S., L.D.N., R.D., and
Joan Clark, M.S., R.D., C.D.E.

ALPHA

A member of Penguin Group (USA) Inc.

Lucy: To Patrick
Sandy: To my Mom and Dad
Joan: To Jenny, Ryan, and Tricia

ALPHA BOOKS

Published by the Penguin Group

Penguin Group (USA) Inc., 375 Hudson Street, New York, New York 10014, U.S.A.

Penguin Group (Canada), 10 Alcorn Avenue, Toronto, Ontario, Canada M4V 3B2 (a division of Pearson Penguin Canada Inc.)

Penguin Books Ltd., 80 Strand, London WC2R 0RL, England

Penguin Ireland, 25 St Stephen's Green, Dublin 2, Ireland (a division of Penguin Books Ltd.)

Penguin Group (Australia), 250 Camberwell Road, Camberwell, Victoria 3124, Australia (a division of Pearson Australia Group Pty Ltd.)

Penguin Books India Pvt Ltd., 11 Community Centre, Panchsheel Park, New Delhi—110 017, India

Penguin Group (NZ), cnr Airborne and Rosedale Roads, Albany, Auckland 1310, New Zealand (a division of Pearson New Zealand Ltd.)

Penguin Books (South Africa) (Pty) Ltd., 24 Sturdee Avenue, Rosebank, Johannesburg 2196, South Africa

Penguin Books Ltd., Registered Offices: 80 Strand, London WC2R 0RL, England

Copyright © 2005 by Lucy Beale and Sandy G. Couvillon

International Standard Book Number: 1-59257-449-1
Library of Congress Catalog Card Number: 021898574497

07 06   8 7 6 5 4 3 2

Interpretation of the printing code: The rightmost number of the first series of numbers is the year of the book's printing; the rightmost number of the second series of numbers is the number of the book's printing. For example, a printing code of 05-1 shows that the first printing occurred in 2005.

Printed in the United States of America

Note: This publication contains the opinions and ideas of its authors. It is intended to provide helpful and informative material on the subject matter covered. It is sold with the understanding that the authors and publisher are not engaged in rendering professional services in the book. If the reader requires personal assistance or advice, a competent professional should be consulted.

The authors and publisher specifically disclaim any responsibility for any liability, loss, or risk, personal or otherwise, which is incurred as a consequence, directly or indirectly, of the use and application of any of the contents of this book.

Most Alpha books are available at special quantity discounts for bulk purchases for sales promotions, premiums, fundraising, or educational use. Special books, or book excerpts, can also be created to fit specific needs.

For details, write: Special Markets, Alpha Books, 375 Hudson Street, New York, NY 10014.

Publisher: *Marie Butler-Knight*
Editorial Director: *Mike Sanders*
Senior Managing Editor: *Jennifer Bowles*
Acquisitions Editors: *Renee Wilmeth and Michele Wells*
Development Editor: *Nancy D. Lewis*
Production Editor: *Janette Lynn*

Copy Editor: *Kelly D. Henthorne*
Cartoonist: *Shannon Wheeler*
Cover/Book Designer: *Trina Wurst*
Indexer: *Angie Bess*
Layout: *Becky Harmon*
Proofreader: *Donna Martin*

Contents at a Glance

Contents

Foreword

I love this book and you will, too! Lucy Beale's work is the epitome of leading-edge thinking when it comes to reshaping the body and the mind. Lucy and her co-authors, Sandy Couvillon and Joan Clark, reveal the ultimate principles to change your lifestyle and live in your ideal, healthy, and fit body!

I met Lucy Beale in 1998 when I was well over the 300-pound mark. When I say well over, I mean my midriff drifted around my body, covering my hips and resting on my thighs when I sat down. I was not a pretty picture. And I was miserable. I had no self-esteem, hated the body I lived in, and was terribly depressed. Fortunately, somewhere in my brain there was still a cell that believed I could overcome obesity, and that cell somehow found Lucy Beale ... just like you have found this book.

Lucy taught me to stop telling myself I was fat when I awoke every morning, to start being kind to myself, and, most importantly, to begin communicating immediately with my body. I had never heard of the 0-to-5 hunger scale, and this ingenious strategy taught me to get in touch with my body. After a few months of using Lucy's philosophy, I called her up and told her, "Lucy, I have never really lived in my body!"

When I was overweight, I always felt empty and kept feeding the feeling. That feeling of emptiness was my body and mind trying to get my attention! My body was not empty ... it just wasn't fulfilled. In changing my attitudes and behaviors toward food, eating, and my body, I became aware of my body's intelligence. I learned that my body was a great communicator. It always tells me exactly what it wants. My job is to listen and respond responsibly.

The exercise suggestions in the book include some simple ones that have become for me a precious daily gift to my body. Just 10 minutes a day have been enough to help me reach my ideal size and rid myself of a yucky double chin.

Today, several years after adopting Lucy's system, I am five clothing sizes smaller and happier than ever. I used to wear a size 26. Now I wear a size 16. Keeping weight off is no longer the struggle it was in the past.

By following the life-changing principles in this book, you will create a loving relationship with your body. You will want to feed your body just the right amount of wonderful, healthy foods, to take your body for a walk or to a yoga class, and to clothe it in something that reveals its shape! This approach does take some effort, but nothing compared to the struggle of living life as an overweight person. Getting to your ideal size is a life-changing transformation that will make you feel fulfilled, improve your self-esteem, and give you the healthy life you have always desired.

Take this book and devour it! It will be the first time in your life you overindulge in something that will make you naturally thin! I know. I have lived the principles in this book and my reflection in the mirror is one I love!

—Deborah Miles Kelly

Introduction

Yes, you can get to an ideal size that is realistic for you and stay there for life. You can master your eating and your weight. In this book, you will learn how and what to eat, how to think, how to exercise, and how to avoid common weight-loss pitfalls. We won't teach you gimmicky solutions. Instead, you learn the basics that help you lose weight faster and stay healthier. Simple, smart, commonsense approaches are the hallmark of this book.

Start now to plan your new thinner wardrobe and attitude. You can have the results you want and deserve.

How This Book Is Organized

The book is divided into six parts:

Part 1, "What Size Do You Want to Be?" guides you to determine the body size that's best for you. You'll learn about being overweight, the obesity epidemic, and the health risks of excessive weight. Just as important, we'll dispel popular weight myths and replace them with confidence-boosting knowledge, practical advice, and inspiration to get you started on the right path, right away.

Part 2, "Your Basic Weight-Loss Program," introduces you to how your body handles food and eating and what causes it to either gain or lose weight. You will learn to appreciate your body and its appetite, to boost your body's natural metabolic rate, and to avoid the self-defeating starvation metabolism. You'll master simple ways to make eating a relaxed and beautiful part of your life.

Part 3, "Food Supports Your Weight Loss," will give you an understanding of what foods you need for healthy weight loss. You'll read a straightforward explanation of the essential qualities of proteins, fats, and carbohydrates and how you should balance them in your safe, nutritional eating plan. Plus, you'll get valuable insight into using nutritional supplements.

Part 4, "Eating for Weight Loss," gives you guidelines for selecting which of four basic eating plans—low-glycemic, low-carb, low-calorie, or low-fat—is the best for you. You can follow the two-week menus for the plan that best meets your health goals and lifestyle.

Part 5, "Exercise Is Your Friend," explores why exercise is an essential part of developing a healthy body that provides you with a nice body shape, muscle tone, and stamina. We debunk exercise myths and fads and show you how to put together a home program that will help you look good and feel good. You also learn how to incorporate recreational exercise into your lifestyle.

Part 6, "Understanding Weight-Loss Plans," analyzes popular weight-loss plans to steer you to the ones that will work best for you. You'll have a chance to see which ones are gimmicky (maybe even unsafe) and which ones are based on sound principles. We also discuss fad diets and medical approaches.

Part 7, "Get Your Mind-Set Right," uses the principles of the body-mind connection to teach you how visualizations and affirmations can hasten your weight-loss progress. You will learn how to approach dining out, family holidays, and vacations with confidence and ease, knowing that you can continue your progress at all times.

Extra Bites

The sidebars in this book offer tips, inspiration, valuable knowledge, and definitions. Use these as road signs on the journey to your goal—your ideal size.

Lean Lingo

The definitions of words and concepts in these boxes will expand your knowledge of weight loss, nutrition, and health terms ... without expanding your waist.

Thinspiration

Like a friendly weight-loss coach, these boxes contain positive, inspiring, and uplifting thoughts, plus encouragement, for your journey from being overweight to being thin.

Weighty Warning

Mistakes happen, but these warnings should help keep you from stalling your progress and making fattening mistakes.

Body of Knowledge

These facts increase your knowledge base for life-long weight maintenance.

Acknowledgments

Our dream of writing a practical and inspiring guide to weight loss couldn't have become a reality without, first and foremost, our clients and students who have egged us on to find solutions to their weight-loss problems. We appreciate each and every one of you.

Lucy Beale would like to give a special thanks to her loving husband, Patrick Partridge, for his enthusiasm, generous support, and hugs; to Marilyn Allen and Coleen O'Shea for their continual support and enthusiasm for her book projects; and to the online readers of *Lucy's Letter* who continue to inform and inspire her efforts. Lucy thanks her co-authors, Joan and Sandy, for their thoughtful, scientific expertise as well as insightful comments and suggestions while bringing this book to completion.

Joan Clark thanks her children, Jenny, Ryan, and Tricia, for their patience and encouragement. Joan thanks the author, Lucy, for her expertise, enthusiasm, and creativity. She also thanks Dr. Dana Clarke for sharing his expertise on low-glycemic eating and the low-glycemic food guide pyramid.

The authors thank Marilyn Allen of the Allen O'Shea Literary Agency and Renee Wilmeth and Michele Wells, acquisitions editors at Alpha Books, for nurturing this book from inception through publication.

Sandy Couvillon thanks her husband, Brian, for his love and confidence in her. Love and laughter go to her adult children, Courtney and Brad, for years of sampling unfamiliar foods for their "dietitian mom." Much love to her parents, Jim and Velma Guess, who have always believed that she knew her stuff. Sandy appreciates her family for supporting her utmost career desire to educate and impact others with compassion and wisdom. She loves you all dearly.

Finally, we would like to thank you, our reader, because you have acquired this book to help you master your weight. Many of you are frustrated and seeking sound guidance, and we are pleased you have chosen this roadmap on your journey to reach your ideal size. Please let us know when you get there!

Trademarks

Part 1

What Size Do You Want To Be?

If reaching your ideal size and staying there were simple, you wouldn't be reading this book. Nor would we have today's obesity epidemic in the United States. As a nation, we're getting "larger" every year, despite all the low-fat foods, low-carb foods, crash diets, and eating programs we're being asked to buy into. The first part of this book starts you on your journey toward your ideal size by teaching you some fundamental guiding principles.

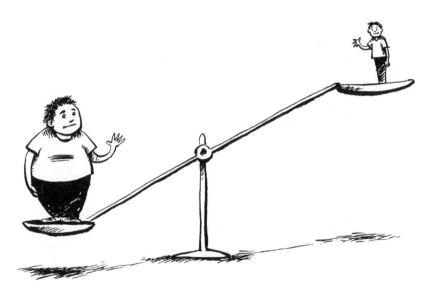

The Joy of Being Your Ideal Size

In This Chapter

- ◆ The U.S. obesity epidemic
- ◆ Health risks of being overweight or obese
- ◆ Knowing you can succeed
- ◆ Very real benefits of living at your ideal size

Picture yourself the way you want to look. That's the image to hold in your head as you read this book. It's also the self-image you should keep for the rest of your life—because that's the way you *can* look!

For now, however, you've got a weight issue. Perhaps you're carrying 15 pounds and a few more inches than your ideal. Maybe it's 50 pounds or more. Perhaps you've tried different diets and food plans, along with various exercise regimes. Most likely, your long-term results have been disappointing. Although you might have lost weight at times, eventually something happened, and you regained the weight, perhaps even more than you lost. Worse, you are at a loss as to why your best efforts have failed.

You know there must be a solution to your weight issue. After all, aren't there plenty of people who both enjoy food and stay at their ideal size, the size that is realistic for them? The good news is that you can be one of them! That's the fundamental message of this book.

A Nation Getting Fatter

Body of Knowledge

The body mass index (BMI) is not a perfect guide, but it's a useful one. There are a few obvious exceptions to the formula: Athletes with very high muscle mass will have a higher BMI, and people, such as the elderly, who have lost a great amount of muscle mass due to reduced nutritional reserves will have a low BMI.

You are not alone. The U.S. population is larger than ever before in history and keeps getting larger. Gradually, we have become a land of "supersized" individuals. More than 67 percent of American adults are overweight and 33 percent are obese. That means more than 97.1 million adults in the United States are unsuccessful at managing their weight.

The medical definition of overweight is having a *body mass index* (BMI) of between 25 and 29.9. If your BMI is between 18.5 and 24.9, you are within the normal weight range. If your BMI is higher than 29.9, you are considered to be obese. To calculate your BMI, multiply your weight in pounds by 704.5, divide the result by your height in inches, and then divide that result by your height in inches a second time. See Chapter 3 for more information on the BMI.

The U.S. population has been getting progressively weightier for the past four decades. The proportion of the population that is overweight or obese has increased from 24.4 percent in 1960 to 67 percent in 2004. Here's how it breaks down:

24.4% in 1960–62
24.9% in 1971–74
25.4% in 1976–80
34.8% in 1988–94
67% in 2004

The trend isn't slowing. The Centers for Disease Control considers obesity to be a frightening medical epidemic. About 20 million men and 20 million women are obese. That's a 61 percent increase since 1991. In 1991, only 4 of 45 states that participated in a National Institute of Health study had obesity rates of 15 to 19 percent of their adult populations. By 2000, 49 of 50 states—Colorado was the one exception—had rates of 15 percent or greater.

What's causing our collective chubbiness? Various pundits place the blame on our sedentary lifestyles, fast food, convenience foods, and processed foods. There simply isn't one cause, nor will a magic pill or potion shrink the population back to size. Being overweight or obese is a condition of lifestyle and poor eating habits, and it can change only when each individual, like you, makes significant and life-enhancing lifestyle changes.

You Can Buck the Trend

Does it make you feel better that so many others are fighting fat, too? Of course it does. Misery loves company, but you're reading this book because you don't want to be part of that crowd. Don't let the statistics discourage you. It might seem inevitable that a person wouldn't have a fighting chance to buck the trend. If everyone is getting fatter, why shouldn't you expect to be overweight also? Because when people change lifestyle and eating habits, they lose weight and keep it off.

Here are five critical and inspirational points to remember as you use this book and lose those pounds:

1. **You get to choose.** Plenty of people—at least 33 percent of the U.S. population—are *not* overweight. You can be one of them. You are not destined to be fat.

2. **You can learn.** You can master the tried-and-true basics of what and how to eat and how to live as a *thin* person.

3. **You can change.** Many formerly overweight people are enjoying the newfound freedom of being their *ideal size* and enjoying food. If they can do it, so can you.

4. **You have the desire.** You obviously have an interest in losing weight. Now you just need to develop the motivation and the wisdom to avoid the fads and the gimmicks that lead to failure.

5. **You can count on us as knowledge-able friends.** In this book, we tell you what works and what doesn't. You're holding in your hands a friendly guide to reach your size goal. We'll show you which exercise and eating changes to make, how to learn from the inevitable mistakes, and how to stay on track for the long term.

Lean Lingo _____

Thin is a loaded word. It means different things to different people. In this book, we use it to describe someone at or near the normal range for BMI. Your **ideal size** is the one that keeps you healthy and makes you happy.

So be confident. The fact that others—many others—are overweight does not predict your fate. Join those who have learned how to eat, what to eat, and how to exercise. Join those who get into their smaller jeans easily. They experience the joy of being free of having a weight problem. So will you.

Your beliefs are a powerful force, so believe you have your ideal body, even though you aren't there already. Believe you are already there. If inconsistent thoughts or actions arise, change them. To create your ideal size, you must create your thoughts and actions accordingly.

Losing Weight Just Ain't What It Used To Be

As recently as 20 years ago, the common thinking about weight loss was simply to eat fewer calories and do more exercise to burn off the calories, and you would easily get to your ideal size. Few people were successful with this formula, and few can be successful using it today. What research shows is that calories overall don't count as much as which foods you eat and how you eat them. We now know that certain foods stimulate hormones that direct weight gain and loss. We know how metabolism works, and we are learning more every day.

Get to Your Ideal Size and Get Healthier

Here's a simple, sobering health fact: thin is healthier; fatter is riskier. The serious health risks associated with being overweight are an alarming aspect of the growing "size" of the U.S. population. The old-fashioned image of a "fat and happy" person belies the jeopardy of chronic health conditions associated with being overweight. Many individuals are familiar with the increased risk of type 2 diabetes, but the problem doesn't stop there. The following are known health risks for being overweight: diabetes (type 2), heart disease, stroke, high blood pressure, gallbladder disease, osteoarthritis and autoimmune disorders, sleep apnea and other breathing problems, cancer (uterine, breast, colorectal, kidney, gallbladder, and endometrial), gout.

Weighty Warning

Almost half of post-menopausal women diagnosed with breast cancer have a body mass index (BMI) equal to or greater than 29. In addition, deaths associated with being overweight now surpass the number of deaths associated with smoking.

Obesity is also associated with the following:

- High cholesterol
- Pregnancy complications
- Menstrual irregularities
- Stress incontinence
- Psychological disorders such as depression
- Increased risk during surgery

Obese individuals have a 50–100 percent increased risk of death from all these causes compared with normal-weight individuals. Perhaps you already have some of these health issues. For example, people who are obese have 30 to 50 percent more chronic medical problems than smokers or problem drinkers.

Get to Your Ideal Size and Enjoy How You Look

You want to look your best. You want to fit into your favorite jeans. You want to make an appearance, turn heads, and receive compliments. You want to feel sensuous and desirable when wearing a swimsuit or going to a party or class reunion. Few of us have the genetics that produce fashion model figures, but we want to have shapes of which we're proud.

Is this the wrong reason to want to be thinner? Would the world be a better place if we all were less vain? Perhaps. But wanting to look your best is a powerful motivator. You can be sure that no naturally thin person is itching to be overweight!

It isn't fun to feel fat in your clothes. It isn't fun to shop for clothing that hides your size. It isn't fun to be physically uncomfortable in airplane seats. It isn't fun to huff and puff up the steps or to avoid health clubs because you're embarrassed by how you look.

Note that we aren't talking about becoming "skinny." ("Skinny" is a word that's hard to define, but somehow we all recognize a truly skinny person.) People who starve themselves to the point of frailty to look pencil-thin are taking serious health risks. This book is *not* about attempting to copy the look of the latest *Vogue* models. It's designed to help you reach your *healthy* ideal size.

Life is challenging enough without being self-conscious about your weight. Later in this book, you will learn to develop the "mindset" of a naturally thin person.

Become More Visible

One of our clients, Mary, commented that the biggest difference for her when she went from a size 18 to a size 8 was that she became "visible." Before, Mary could stand and stand at a cosmetic counter in a big department store and never be helped while those around her were served. Today, the clerks at stores "see" her. They want to sell her cosmetics, clothing, or whatever. At a size 18, Mary was embarrassed to walk into a restaurant and often was ignored. Now when she walks into a restaurant, she is greeted right away, and she feels comfortable and welcome.

You'll become more visible, too, so get familiar with this concept now and plan to enjoy it. Be prepared to accept the responsibility and the resultant delights.

Thinspiration

Right now is a good time to start imagining what it will be like for you to be "visible." Imagine walking into a department store or a restaurant as a trim person. What does it feel like to be noticed? Some people who lose weight find it somewhat scary and intimidating to be "seen." Prepare yourself now. Just for fun, the next time you enter a nice restaurant dressed appropriately, imagine being "visible" like a famous movie star. Make an entrance. Let yourself feel glamorous. If you think it would be too hard to actually do this, let your imagination play out the fantasy.

Look Forward to More Romance

It's probably fortunate that romantic attraction between men and women is more mystery and magic than science. We are attracted to each other for a host of reasons, and physical looks is only one of them. But physical attraction based on looks is certainly very real.

Feeling desirable can have a direct effect on the quality of your romantic life. By contrast, feeling fat can hinder one's love life. Being perceived as fat hinders it even more.

Sadly, this is true even in long-term, loving relationships. Physical attraction can diminish when one or both partners become overweight. Should you be angry about it? No! Go ahead and focus on romance now by making yourself as desirable as possible at your current size. Then proceed to get to your ideal size ... and look forward to enjoying extra sizzle in your romantic life.

Get to Your Ideal Size and Join In on Financial Rewards

Get rid of the excess inches by depositing them in the bank! Okay, you can't literally do that, but there are often professional and income benefits from reaching your ideal size. Over time, the extra income can add considerably to your net worth.

Workplace discrimination against overweight people is seldom discussed and certainly not openly acknowledged, but you know it's there. You may have been told in some ambiguous way that, if you don't lose weight, you will be passed over for promotion or, even worse, will be downsized. ("Downsized" is not a happy word in this context.) Perhaps you have already been derailed or knocked out of the running for a promotion and pay increase while a less-qualified-but-thinner colleague got the job you deserved. You may never be able to prove you were discriminated against, but you know.

Yes, this is illegal, and it's infuriating. In its most blatant forms, it's obnoxious and even immoral. But that doesn't make it less real. Many clients have recounted sad stories of such job discrimination. We hope that weight discrimination will decrease over time, but don't count on it happening soon.

The real problem may be much more subtle. Those who discriminate may be doing so entirely subconsciously. Research by John Cawley of the University of Michigan has shown that a white woman who is perceived as being overweight may earn 7 percent less in pay than a woman who is perceived to be at her ideal size. In a 40-year work career with an estimated annual salary of $30,000, the average overweight woman can lose $84,000 in earning power. Think about how many vacations and pairs of shoes that money could buy!

If you are in a profession in which you have direct contact with customers and the public, your perceived size can make a big difference in your performance and pay. Why? Because you are subject to people's underlying prejudices about overweight individuals—even if they are overweight themselves. Many professional salespersons, especially women, who are at their ideal size earn more than those who are overweight.

What is a person to do? Get to your ideal size and stay there. If you're a woman, you may be giving yourself a 7 percent raise. By the way, this doesn't mean you need to accept the prejudice or the implicit underlying assumptions that prejudiced people make. The assumptions aren't kind, noble, or loving, but we all have irrational prejudices. Get to your ideal size for personal reasons and, in the process, attain your professional and personal goals and ensuing rewards. Then, when you're in a position of authority, make sure that you never, never discriminate against someone with a weight issue … because you've been there yourself.

Get to Your Ideal Size and Enjoy Life More

Losing weight most likely has been one of your major lifetime projects. Certainly, it has taken time and energy. You've learned about nutrition and various diets and food systems. You've succeeded at times and failed most of the time. You might have worked at your weight issues endlessly and worried thousands of hours about your size, your eating, and your behaviors. As you get to your ideal size, you will free up time and energy that can be used more constructively.

Lose Weight, Find Time

What would happen if much of your weight-management time and energy were put into more uplifting, positive, and satisfying activities? What would happen if you didn't need to constantly diet or worry whether your clothes will fit? How would your life change?

Here's a short quiz to take. Write down your honest answers:

- ◆ How many times a day do you think about your weight?

  _____

- ◆ How often do you step on the scale in a week?

  _____

- ◆ How much time do you spend thinking about which foods are "okay"?

  _____

- ◆ How much time do you spend figuring out how to dress in ways that hide your size?

  _____

- ◆ How often do you feel guilty for eating a particular food?

  _____

- ◆ How many times have you wondered what others thought about your size?

  _____

- ◆ How many hours in your lifetime have you stood looking in the mirror examining your hips and thighs?

  _____

◆ Do you think someone who has naturally thin habits spends his or her time doing these things?

_____

◆ What would you rather be doing with your time and energy?

_____

Your weight management won't be one of the most significant contributions you make in your life. Your size will not be written about in your obituary. You have more important things to do in life than deal with a weight issue. So make this the last time you put energy and effort into weight loss. Now is the time.

Thinspiration

Make a list of what you would do if you were already at your ideal size. Then either do these things or make plans to do them.

Mastering Your Weight

You are the only person who can master your body's weight. Only you get to vote on your size. You determine your success. No one else can do it for you.

By mastering your eating and your size, you …

◆ Understand your body and its needs.

◆ Know which foods and nutrition work best for you.

◆ Do exercises that make you feel good and look good.

◆ Understand your individual metabolism and how to boost it.

◆ Stay healthier and avoid overweight-related health problems.

◆ Stay at your ideal size throughout your lifetime.

◆ Sensuously enjoy food and eating.

◆ Remain in charge of your eating, your size, and your weight.

◆ Set a good example for your children.

Affirm your life's purpose. Dieting isn't it, and neither is overeating. If you aren't sure what it is, pretend you know. Tell yourself, "I am now fulfilling my life's purpose."

The Least You Need to Know

◆ The number of overweight and obese people has reached national epidemic proportions.

◆ By getting to your ideal size, you'll improve your health and reduce health risks associated with being overweight and obese.

◆ Generally speaking, women who are at their ideal size earn more income than women who are overweight.

◆ You can begin to enjoy the benefits of looking good and feeling good right now.

◆ As you master your weight, you will free up your energy for more creative and productive pursuits.

2

What Prevents Weight Loss

In This Chapter

- ◆ Internal and external barriers to weight loss
- ◆ Health factors in weight loss
- ◆ Predispositions to being overweight
- ◆ Changing your weight-loss assumptions

Why is weight loss so difficult? You tackle many problems every day that seem much more challenging—your job, family life, budgets, even just driving a car through traffic. What makes shedding inches and keeping them off so prone to failure?

You already have a weight-loss history of what works and doesn't work for you. You probably also have some prejudices that might not be valid. In this chapter, we give you fresh insights about yourself, both physical and mental. You'll learn to approach losing weight realistically and to determine what can be changed, what can be enhanced, and what needs to be accepted.

Death, Taxes, and Body Shape

Just as death and taxes are inevitable, some aspects of your body condition are inevitable, too. You cannot change them, but you can make the best of them. They seem like barriers to achieving your ideal size, but they don't have to be. They are as follows: aging, genetics, hormones, menopause (for women), middle-age spread (for both men and women), and childbirth (for women).

The Aging Weight Myth

There is a popular myth about aging and weight that goes like this: as you get older, you get bigger. It's only a myth. You don't need to get bigger as you age. Plenty of older people have great bodies and enjoy eating and stay at their ideal size. Remember, all you need is one example of a myth not being true to know that it doesn't need to be true for you.

Does age affect body size and shape at all? Of course. In general, as we age, our metabolism naturally slows down. A slower metabolism means we burn calories more slowly. So, eating less food helps to avoid weight gain. But you can also keep your metabolism high through strength training and eating well nutritionally. We'll cover this in much greater detail later in the book.

Your Genes Don't Come from a Designer

You'll have to be content without designer "genes." The genes passed down from your ancestors through your biological parents are yours forever, good and bad. You cannot change your genetics. But you can learn to make the most of what you've been given. (Yes, researchers are seeking the "fat" gene, but they still haven't found one that absolutely predicts obesity.)

Some aspects of heredity affect your body shape, but your genes alone can't make you fat. They determine your basic shape and height as well as your musculature. But heredity is only one of many factors that affect your shape and size.

An old adage tells us: if your parents and relatives are overweight, you will also be overweight. If you come from a "large" family, this can seem to be true. However, think back for a moment to how your family ate. What size portions did they expect you to eat? Were you required to clean your plate before you ate a treat, meaning dessert? Did the family center all celebrations around food and lots of it? Were you taught at an early age to seek out food for solace, celebration, and reward? Maybe it's not your genetics dictating your size but your family's attitude toward food and eating.

Behaviors in "fat" families are more likely to predict overweight offspring than genetics. You can, however, learn new eating habits. You can leave food on your plate; you can become a picky eater; and you can send your leftover food right down the garbage disposal. Isn't that what a garbage disposal is for?

In Chapter 28, you'll learn how to eat at family gatherings and have fun without overindulging … all while staying at your ideal size.

Aagh! Those Raging Hormones!

Hormones often get the blame for everything from obesity to thick thighs. Have you ever said to yourself, "If it weren't for my hormones, I would be able to lose this weight?" You're right in part, but only in part. Hormonal systems that are out of balance can wreak havoc on your weight-loss dreams. You could experience a slower metabolism, weight gain around your midsection, insulin resistance, and water retention, to name a few.

You have, however, considerable power to change your hormonal balance. A combination of proper and delicious nutrition, specific exercises (such as the five Tibetan exercises in Part 5), and plenty of sunshine on a regular basis can help keep your hormones in balance while freeing up excess stored fat.

You may have hormonal imbalances due to the surgical removal of glands such as the thyroid or ovaries. Replacement medications help. Work with your doctor to adjust your dosage so that you feel your best and have the most energy possible. Hormones definitely affect your weight, but you are not stuck with "bad" hormones. Your lifestyle makes a big difference.

> **Lean Lingo**
>
> **Hormones** are made within the body to stimulate and regulate cellular and glandular functions. **Perimenopause** is the 10–12 year transition leading up to menopause. During this time the body's hormone production and metabolic rate slow down.

Menopause Isn't a Menace

As a woman gets to the age of about 50 (give or take), she goes through the change of life, or menopause. This process starts as early as age 30 with *perimenopause*. Her body changes in many ways as the production of estrogen slows down. Menstrual periods cease; metabolism slows; and the skin gets thinner.

Unfortunately, plenty of myths about menopause abound, such as menopause being a time when a woman can expect to gain weight. As inevitable as menopause is, it doesn't have to go hand in hand with weight gain. Yes, some women gain weight at this time, usually because their metabolism is slower and they're eating the same amount of food as they did at age 25.

But if a woman eats just the amount of food that her body needs for fuel, eats nutrient-packed foods, and exercises for both strength and stamina, she can stay at her ideal size with ease.

In other words, menopause is a fact of life. It is not an excuse for being overweight.

That Useless Spare Tire

Men tend to carry "spare tires" around their waist come middle age. All the crunches at the gym don't seem to help much. In fact, a man can have terrifically strong stomach muscles and still have a larger waist and midsection.

The spare tire is often caused by stress. Adrenaline is the "fight or flight" hormone you secrete during stress from normal daily events such as driving, working, and so on. The more stress you experience, the more adrenal hormones your body excretes. One stress hormone, cortisol, causes the body to store fat specifically around the waist. So the more stress, the more cortisol production, the more waist. Can this be changed? Yes, in several ways: through eating nutritiously so that you get plenty of stress-busting nutrients, by doing those crunches with complementary stretching, and by decompressing everyday.

When "Baby Fat" Isn't on the Baby

Many women complain they never lost the weight they gained during pregnancy. Of course, a woman naturally weighs more during pregnancy and even up to a year after childbirth. She's biologically programmed to gradually release her "baby" weight during the first year after birth. Some women, however, don't lose the weight. This can be caused by hormones and also because the women continue to eat as they did when pregnant.

Weighing more during pregnancy is a fact of life. Not being able to lose the "baby" fat doesn't have to be. Your youthful shape can return just as it has for many other women. By using the nutritional guidelines in Part 3 of this book, you'll give your body the support it needs.

But I Love Food!

Yes, you do love food. Hooray! Biologically, you are designed to love food. Of course, some food lovers are at their ideal size, and some aren't. Your confusion about your love of food could be getting in the way of reaching your ideal size. Do any of the following sound familiar?

"If it weren't for chocolate." Chocolate is delicious and enticing. It tastes good. It makes us feel good. You don't need to give up your chocolate to lose weight. In fact, you shouldn't. Dark chocolate is brimming with antioxidants and is good for your health. Just don't overdo it. Eat chocolate slowly and savor every taste sensation. Don't deny yourself the foods you love—that could lead you to binge later.

"If it weren't for (you fill in the blank)." Perhaps you've read that certain foods make you fat, and you think they contribute to your weight problem. Any food can make you fat, and any food can make you thin, depending on how you eat it. The good news is that there aren't evil foods. You can eat all foods and still reach your ideal size. This doesn't mean you can overeat these foods or binge on them. Eat them normally, enjoy them, and let them give you nutrition, pleasure, and energy, which is what food is for.

"If it weren't for fast food." Let's face it. Fast food is part of our lives. It's quick, easy, inexpensive, and sustains us, at least temporarily. You can eat fast food once in a while and lose weight. "Once in a while" is the operative phrase here. In Chapter 26, we show you how to eat at fast-food restaurants while getting to your ideal size.

> **Thinspiration**
>
> One of the wonderful things about losing weight is that you lose weight by eating, not by avoiding food or starving yourself. Your love of food and enjoyment of it can propel you to your ideal size. What a delight—the very thing that caused your weight gain is the very thing that will bring you success.

Other People and Your Eating

Other people in your life can seem to derail your weight-loss success. Perhaps you have thought that if you didn't have them around, especially at mealtime, you could easily master your weight. The reality, however, is this: those people *are* part of your life. You can be thin regardless of your relationships with others, and in Chapter 27, we tell you how.

Cooking and Your Eating

You may be cooking meals for a family, including growing children with racecar metabolisms. They may be able to eat masses of spaghetti and never gain an ounce. You not only have to cook for them and eat with them, you are in agony while you watch them devour food.

You can master this situation. The basic guideline is this: eat the same foods they eat, just not the same quantity. Yes, you can enjoy pizza. You do not need to eat special foods or make a big deal with your family about your diet. You can confidently eat with them and lose weight.

Eating and Your Relationships

Do any of these sound familiar. If only I didn't have to eat with my spouse; if only I weren't in a relationship; if only I were in a relationship; if only I didn't have to feed my children ….

Actually, none of these statements has much to do with what or how you eat, but you might think they do. If you're trying to keep up with another person bite for bite, forkful for forkful, it won't be a "losing" situation.

The late comedian Flip Wilson, imitating a child, would get laughs with his "The devil made me do it!" excuse for being bad. It didn't work for the child, and it won't work for you. We doubt someone is opening your mouth and force-feeding you, so forget trying to place blame elsewhere.

You can learn the skills to eat with others while you lose weight. The simple rules for eating to lose weight are the same regardless of with whom you eat. As you learn to enjoy eating again, you'll rediscover the joys of eating with others—the camaraderie, the interesting conversations, the laughter, the sharing. Dining with others is one of the good parts of life.

Weight Is a Time Issue

It takes time to lose weight. Time as measured in months or years, but also in the clock time it takes. If you want to know what you love, notice where you put your time. If you don't take the time to lose weight, it isn't a high-enough priority.

Remember, worrying about your weight takes time, too. If you devote time now to reaching your ideal size, you'll save time in the long run.

Exercise, Time, and You

No one has time to exercise. Who has time to take off during a busy day and spend 30 to 45 minutes sweating and huffing and puffing? You do. How do we know? Because we know this: if exercise is important to you, you'll find a way. If you have enough time to watch just one television show, you have time to exercise.

Besides, exercise isn't about time; it's about love. The love of health, well-being, energy, and vitality. It's about your commitment to life at your ideal size. You know this.

Body of Knowledge
Here's a time guideline to attaining your ideal size. Figure that it takes about two to three months to lose a dress size or belt size. You may lose your weight more quickly, but use this guide for planning.

Cooking, Time, and You

Few people have enough time anymore to cook beautiful meals, so prepare delicious meals that feature simplicity and good nutrition. Getting the nutrition you need to lose weight doesn't require lots of cooking time. It requires thoughtfulness and care. Having time to cook is not a requirement for losing weight.

Fortunately, you don't need to cook to lose weight. It makes no difference whether you cook at home, have others cook for you, eat out, or eat takeout. Your size is independent of your attitude toward cooking. As an example, you can eat raw, fresh foods. You can purchase healthy, ready-made foods from delicatessens and salad bars. Most grocery stores have interesting takeout sections.

Cook stunning meals if you want, but don't sweat it if you and the stove are not on a first-name basis.

Medical Conditions

If you have a medical condition that gets in the way of losing weight, learn how to make the best of your health situation. Certain medical conditions can definitely slow down your weight loss, but don't let them stop or thwart your efforts.

Low Thyroid

An underactive thyroid gland can suppress your metabolism and keep your weight on. Your best bet is to fine-tune your dosage of thyroid medication with your doctor's assistance. If you suspect that your thyroid is out of balance, make sure that your doctor assesses all aspects of your thyroid production:

 ◆ T3, which is the stronger of the two key hormones produced by the thyroid gland and is also produced from the conversion of T4.

 ◆ T4, which is the primary hormone produced by the thyroid gland.

 ◆ TSH, which is the hormone produced by the pituitary gland that stimulates the thyroid gland. Measurement of TSH is considered a primary way to diagnose thyroid disorders.

Some people respond better on a combination of T3 and T4; some do fine on T4 alone.

Some clients do best on regular prescription meds for thyroid support. Others do best with natural thyroid medications such as Armour. You can also use alternative health support, such as naturally compounded thyroid, homeopathic remedies, and the ayurvedic herbal extract, forslean.

Daily exercise helps to balance your hormones. Be sure to take 5 to 10 minutes every day to do the Tibetan exercises in Part 4.

Some Medications

Several medications can prevent weight loss or cause you to gain weight. Steroids virtually always cause weight gain. Even asthma inhalers contain enough steroids to slow or stop your progress. Talk with your doctor and ask him or her to suggest alternatives to your current steroid medications. Also ask what you can do to ease off them.

Some psychotropic and anti-seizure drugs can also affect your weight. Most often these cause weight loss, but some (such as Depakote) can cause weight gain. Again, ask your doctor to work with you to find one that does not affect your weight.

Pain

Chronic pain can inhibit your desire to exercise. If you are in continual pain from injuries or arthritis, you could also be using food to soothe the pain. Be sure you make other choices for pain relief. Certainly, it can be difficult to do much exercise with severe or chronic pain, but it is possible to do *some* exercise. Get the advice of a physical therapist or specialist to find exercises that are healing for you.

Whenever you become inactive, for whatever reason, your body needs less food than before. Often people do not adjust their food intake when they become inactive, and they gain weight. If you are currently inactive, reduce the amount of food you are eating to accommodate your inactivity and the resulting slower metabolism.

Low Blood Sugar

Low blood sugar happens when your blood sugar drops fast and catches you unaware. At such times, you may experience headaches, nausea, irritability, crankiness, and a lightheaded feeling. You also get heavy-duty cravings for food—any kind of food and lots of it.

Low blood sugar can result in bingeing or overeating sweet, starchy foods such as cookies, cakes, crackers, and breads. The key to tackling a low-blood-sugar condition is to eat enough protein and fat at meals. Plus, keep snacks around—in your handbag or desk—and eat them when you feel like you're running on empty. By using the nutritional advice in this book, low blood sugar can become an aspect of your past and not your present.

Diabetes

Diabetes and weight gain share an unfortunate symbiotic relationship. Sixty-seven percent of adults with Type 2 diabetes have a BMI of 27 or higher, which means they're overweight. Type 2 diabetes was once called *adult onset diabetes* because a person is not born with it; rather, you develop it as an adult. Diabetes in children has increased ten-fold in the past 20 years, so the term, adult onset diabetes, has been dropped. People who are overweight or obese are at high risk of developing this disease. If for no other reason, you should get your weight down to reduce your risk.

Type 2 diabetics who regulate their blood-sugar levels with diet and not with insulin can often more easily reach their ideal size. If you are using insulin to control blood-sugar levels, approach any weight-loss program carefully with close monitoring of your blood-sugar levels. That way, you'll avoid insulin levels that are too high. Too much insulin in the body causes weight gain.

> CAUTION
>
> **Weighty Warning** _____
>
> The rate of Type 2 diabetes in the United States is skyrocketing, partially due to the increase in obesity. More than 18.2 million adults—or 6.3 percent of the U.S. population—have Type 2 diabetes. If you already have Type 2 diabetes, the closer you get to your ideal size, the more likely it is that your health will improve. If you don't have diabetes, reaching your ideal size will lower your risk for having this health condition.

Birth Control Pills

Birth control pills have been known to cause weight gain—sometimes a little, sometimes a lot—in many women. Fortunately, the hormone dosage in today's birth control pills is lower than ever before and should not be a big factor in weight gain. With that said, however, you could still be gaining weight by using them. If this is the case, talk with your doctor to find a formulation that reduces weight gain.

The birth control shots and systems that last for three months at a time are more problematic. They can wreak havoc with your hormones and add on the pounds. Think carefully about whether the three-month formulations are worth the weight. Yes, they're convenient, but are they necessary? Find another method if you are battling an increase in weight while using this method.

You Can Master These Weight-Loss Barriers

Certain barriers to weight loss are easy to change. Doing your part from a lifestyle point of view can work wonders. In fact, sometimes making only one change can assist you in shedding pounds.

Enjoy Your Beauty Rest

Are you getting enough vitamin ZZZZ? You need adequate sleep. If you're deprived of sleep regularly, you'll struggle to reach your ideal size. Remember the saying "If you snooze, you lose"? Well, hooray! With weight loss, it's true! Research has shown that if you don't snooze, you gain.

Figuring out how much sleep you need is the question. You require basically the same amount of sleep per night every night. Chances are, the amount you need has remained fairly constant throughout most of your life. You probably need somewhere between six and nine hours of sleep every night.

Don't fret if your sleep needs are on the high end. It's not a "badge of honor" to get by on less sleep. This "getting by" attitude is fattening. During sleep, your body relaxes and releases fat. Without enough sleep, your body's cortisol levels climb and your stress levels are higher, making your body hoard fat.

Plan your life so that you get the sleep your body requires. Yes, some nights you won't get enough sleep, but make them infrequent. Remember, those thin jeans are going to feel so good when they finally fit.

Too Much Fight-or-Flight Adds Pounds

Living a life of continual high stress keeps you fat and can actually increase your weight. Adrenaline is our friend when we need it for emergencies, but it was never intended to be tapped on a day-to-day basis to deal with traffic, anxiety, work-related issues, and deadlines. If you live with stressful deadlines, a high-stress job, a frantic daily commute, and so forth, losing weight will be an uphill battle ... and another source of stress!

Your best choice for dealing with continual stress is to schedule time periods when you simply relax. Don't run errands, paint the bedroom, or clean out the garage. Instead, snuggle on the sofa with a good read. Rent funny movies and enjoy some laughs. Give yourself the luxury of really resting, and by the next morning, you may just find that your jeans are looser.

Here's another example: ever wonder why you sometimes lose weight on vacation? It could be that your body is off the adrenaline rush long enough to release fat stores it doesn't need. If you vacation infrequently, make a habit of taking a whole day off whenever you can. Then do nothing productive. Amazing, isn't it? Thin and lazy sometimes go together!

The Dark Side of Caffeine

A good cup of coffee is certainly a delight and, for some people, is pretty much a necessity for getting the day started. Perhaps you even drink a cup or two mid-afternoon to perk up from an energy slump. The same could be said for tea, caffeinated soda, and diet sodas. Caffeine is tricky. It can prevent you from losing weight and can contribute to weight gain.

How can this be? Caffeine has no calories. But calories are not the only factor in weight loss. Caffeine stimulates the pancreas to, in a sense, overproduce insulin. Insulin is one of your hormones that cause your body to store fat.

Does this mean you should never have a cup of coffee again? Not really. You don't need to give up caffeine, but you could benefit by changing the way you drink caffeinated beverages. The simple rule of thumb is this: have your caffeinated beverage _with_ a meal, not before a meal or all by itself. (By the way, putting cream and sugar in coffee or tea does not count as a meal.) By having food with your beverage, the insulin is not overproduced; it's more balanced.

It is also perfectly fine to give up caffeine entirely. Plenty of people do. They seem to function fine, although their caffeinated friends find this hard to believe. If you want to get off coffee or caffeine, you can wean yourself off slowly or go "cold turkey." In either case, expect to be physically uncomfortable for a while. The most common reactions are lethargy and headaches. They go away after several days to a week.

Allergies Add Pounds

Eating foods that you are allergic to or sensitive to will work against your best efforts at weight loss. If you're allergic to a food or are highly sensitive to it and you go ahead and eat it anyway, you'll pay the price. When you ingest a known allergen, the body gets defensive. It uses several strategies for dealing with allergens: it bloats; it refuses to digest; it might push the food through the digestive tract too quickly; it creates mucous to prevent nutrients from being absorbed in the intestines; it can wad the food into a ball in your bowel and refuse to dispel it. The body does many things with such a food—except use it for nutrition.

Many foods that cause allergies and sensitivities are common foods that are widely available and seem to be in everything edible. The most difficult to eliminate from your diet include wheat, corn, soy, and dairy.

If you suspect that you're allergic to a specific food, you can get verification from a skin test given at an allergist's office. In the meantime, give up the food. Some chiro-practors and alternative health practitioners can also test for food allergies and sensi-tivities.

A Little Taste of Sweet

If you make a habit of sipping on sweet liquids—even artificially sweetened ones—throughout the day, you may have difficulty losing weight. Ditto eating mints or bits of candy throughout the day. This isn't really about the calories you ingest; it's more about how the sweet taste works with the digestive system.

When the tongue tastes something sweet, the body assumes that it's going to be receiving food and nutrients. It then begins to store the food it is currently digesting, turning that food into fat. After all, the body won't need the energy from the food already in the digestive process if more is on the way. The digestive system doesn't know that it's only going to get a bit of something sweet. It just does as it's programmed—it stores fat.

So, how are you going to drink sweet-tasting liquids like juice or a beverage sweetened with sugar or an artificial sweetener? Hopefully, you'll pass on the artificial sweeteners—they've been shown to thwart weight loss. Drink sweetened beverages and juice with meals or snacks. Fortunately, you don't need to be stuck with an impossible weight issue. Today, with medical advances and common sense, there are excellent solutions for tough weight-loss concerns.

> **Thinspiration**
>
> Sip on water during the day as an alternative to sipping on sweet drinks. Sweet drinks, including all diet drinks, confuse the body. Water has terrific therapeutic and health benefits. Your body loves water.

The Least You Need to Know

- Virtually all body conditions that prevent weight loss can be remedied.
- Review your reasons for not being able to lose weight and resolve to either correct them or let them go.
- Do what is necessary to clear up any body conditions that have kept your weight on.
- Work with your health professionals to correct medical conditions that can prevent weight loss.

Chapter 3

Choosing Your Ideal Size

In This Chapter

♦ Choosing the size that feels best to you

♦ Selecting your ideal clothing size

♦ Measuring your body fat percentage and BMI

♦ Establishing your attainable goals

You have embarked on a journey to lose weight and get to your ideal size. You need to know your destination. Where do you want to end up? What size will mark the end of your journey? When you select your ideal size, remember that if you don't like it when you get there, you can choose a different size.

Your ideal size is the size that feels the best, at which you have the most energy, the best health, and the highest self-confidence and self-esteem. In this chapter, you will learn several methods for determining your ideal size. We recommend simple strategies but also have included the preferred medical ways to select your size.

Beware the Scales

Thank goodness, scales are finally out of favor. More and more people and professionals understand the limitations of scales and are finding other methods for measuring body size.

A scale doesn't really tell you much that you don't already know, but for a perfectly harmless device in itself, a scale sure can alter a person's moods. If you get on a scale in the morning and have lost a pound, you can feel great about yourself all day. Inside, however, you may be wondering why it wasn't two pounds. If you have stayed at the same weight as the day before, you are doing fine, but on second thought, not all that well. If the scale reads more than yesterday, you feel like a failure, get depressed, and question the validity of your diet and your self-discipline. You probably also will question the accuracy of the scale! By the end of the day, you can descend into a dire sense of failure that cries out for food, glorious food, to soothe your lowered sense of self-esteem.

Scales scientifically measure your specific gravity in relationship to the earth. That's all. They do not tell you how you look or how much body fat you have. They don't measure what's truly going on inside your body. They only measure your weight at a very specific point in time; they tell you nothing about how you fit into your clothes. But try explaining that logic to a person who compulsively visits the scale six to eight times a day.

A woman who has plenty of healthy muscle mass may appear to be the same size as a woman who has a high percentage of body fat. Who weighs more? The first woman weighs more because muscle weighs more than fat. A cubic inch of muscle weighs more than a cubic inch of fat. Every cubic inch of fat you release and every cubic inch of muscle you gain will make you look thinner, although your weight may not go down.

As you do the strength-training exercises in this book to increase your muscle tone and shape, you could end up weighing more than your goal—and looking better than your goal.

One middle-aged male client, Bill, came to his fifth class session delighted that he needed to purchase a new belt. He had lost about 5 to 6 inches from his waist, but he lamented that he hadn't lost any weight at all. What happened? Bill's new exercise regime and eating patterns resulted in lost inches. Many inches. The weight on the scale was not relevant. He was already at the *size* he wanted.

It might feel scary to not step on the scale daily. Get over it. If the scale is too tempting, put it in cold storage and haul it out once a year for an annual "weigh-in."

How Do Your Jeans Fit?

Jeans are rather unforgiving. They don't have an elastic waistband (at least, we hope they don't). They aren't made from some stretchy knit fabric designed to let you grow unhindered and unobserved. They are denim, rugged and classic denim. They don't budge for your bulges.

Do you have a favorite pair of jeans that you've saved because they once fit? Do you secretly long for the day when you can zip them up comfortably and know you look great? Save those jeans. They are your benchmark for how you are doing with your weight loss. Keep them for the rest of your life.

Now that you're heading toward your ideal size, try on your old favorite jeans every month or so. The jeans cannot lie. They're always the same size. As you progress toward your ideal size, you will easily see the progress you are making. When you finally fit into them, it's a real "hurrah!" moment, one you will savor and use for continual inspiration.

Using the jeans method for determining your ideal size means you don't need to weigh in. Of course, it's not a scientific measurement. Do you care? If you need a target number, you might need another measuring stick. But many people who are already thin use this method to stay at their ideal size. The instant their jeans are tight, they are careful about food intake for a couple of days or weeks until their jeans once again fit comfortably.

Jeans make you feel sexy. They are youthful, fun, and speak loudly and proudly of your weight-loss success.

Lean Lingo

Whatever ideal size you choose, affirm you are that size frequently throughout your day. Say, "I now wear a size (insert your ideal size)." Say it even if you aren't at that weight yet. This may sound nuts to you. That's okay. Say it anyway. Affirm your ideal size as often as you think about it. This activity will propel you toward your goal.

What's in a Size?

Clothing sizes are an imprecise but highly effective guide to measuring your weight-loss success. If you're a woman, pick a dress size that you would like to wear. If you want to shop the size-8 racks, make them your target and imagine yourself doing just that. Go for it. You may find yourself picking a smaller dress-size goal after you've reached your first one.

One of our class participants, Marian, who is in her early 50s, made up a mantra that she said to herself often, "It's never too late to be an 8." Upon reaching that goal, she wrote yet another mantra with the assistance of her son Michael, "It's the kicks to be a 6." Within several months, Marian was buying size 6 shorts—a size she never thought possible when she was a size 12.

Women usually think of size in terms of dress size, men in terms of their belt size. So, fellows, if you want a waist size of 34, 36, or whatever, select the one that feels best to you. Using the select-a-size method to choose your ideal size is not particularly scientific, but it's a good measure for how you look—and no scale is needed. It works for many people. Before you select your ideal size for certain, you need to learn about your frame size.

The Frame You Were Born With

The size of your body frame gives a good indication of what clothing size would work best for you. Body frames come in three general sizes: small, medium, and large. A person's frame size doesn't change over a lifetime, just as the color of one's eyes doesn't change. Regardless of the size of your frame, you can get to a clothing size that feels good to you.

> **Body of Knowledge**
>
> Here is how to determine your body frame size. Take your dominant hand. Encircle the wrist of your nondominant hand with the middle finger and thumb. If your middle finger and thumb overlap, you have a small frame. If they just touch, you have a medium frame. If they don't touch, you have a large frame.

A woman with a small frame can wear a smaller size because her hipbones are closer together. She could be comfortable at a size 6 or 8, perhaps a 10. With a medium frame, a woman might choose to be a size 8, 10, or 12. With a large frame, perhaps she would choose a size 10, 12, or 14, depending upon her height. Although a size 14 could sound like a large size to you, we have plenty of clients who look terrific and thin at that size. Your dress size is actually less important than how you look in your clothes and the state of your health at that size.

Hollywood press releases and glamour magazines tell us that some of our favorite movie and television actresses wear a size 0 or 2. You may be wondering how this is possible. Many people who are highly photogenic—think high-fashion models and screen stars—have tiny little faces. Generally speaking, they have very small body frames. Their hipbones are quite close together, and they can wear very small sizes.

These people are genetically unusual—they simply aren't like most of us. Don't worry about it. It's important that you are comfortable and content with the frame size you were born with and make the most of it.

Fat and Muscle Weight Are Quite Different

Another significant measure of body size is body fat percentage. The higher your body fat percentage, the more at risk you are for health issues related to being over-weight or obese. When you have your body fat tested at a health club or at the doctor's, the machine gives you a reading of body fat, water, and muscle percentages. All three add up to 100 percent. Assuming that the amount of water weight remains almost constant for each individual, the variables are body fat and muscle. The more muscle you have, the less body fat you have (and vice versa). Muscle weighs three times more than fat.

Here are ideal body fat percentages:

Women:	Up to age 20	14–21%
	Age 20 to 50	17–27%
	Age 50+	20–30%
Men:	Up to age 20	9–15%
	Age 20 to 50	14–21%
	Age 50+	19–23%

In body fat measurements, lower is not necessarily better. A person must have at least some body fat to be healthy. Fat pads internal organs such as the kidneys, and it also offers protection against cold weather. For women, the minimum recommended fat percentage is 12 percent. If a woman has less, her menstrual cycles could cease. Men must have a minimum of 5 percent to stay healthy.

As you lose weight and do strength-building exercises, your body fat percentage goes down, and your muscle mass increases. This is good because having more muscle gives you the following:

- More physical stamina

- More energy

- A higher metabolic rate

- Better muscle definition

- Better shape (for guys, muscle definition; for gals, curves)

- Higher weight as measured on a scale

- Lower risk of diseases associated with being overweight or obese

A high percentage of body fat is not good. More body fat puts you at a higher risk for diabetes and other medical conditions associated with being overweight or obese, such as high blood pressure, elevated triglyceride levels, metabolic syndrome, cancers, autoimmune disorders, and heart disease. In addition, you will have less energy, a slower metabolic rate, and a flabby body.

Using body fat percentage as a method to measure your ideal size can be misleading. It's part of the picture, but it's not the total picture. One client, Susie, had a body fat reading of only 19 percent. She wore a size 10. However, her waist was quite thick, and her muscles were so large that she didn't like how she looked in clothes. Her jeans didn't fit. Her body fat percentage was ideal, but she still was a larger size than she wanted. Susie needed to eat and exercise differently. Consider using body fat as one measure of your goal, but not the only measure.

Thinspiration

By doing strength-training exercises for as little as six months at two to three hours a week, you can reduce your body fat percentage by as much as 10 percentage points.

The Professional Choice—BMI

Health and medical professionals use the body mass index (BMI) to determine whether you are overweight or obese. The formula figures both weight and height together but doesn't take into account body fat percentage or muscle mass. You need to know your weight in pounds to use the chart that follows.

						BMI (kg/m²)								
	19	**20**	**21**	**22**	**23**	**24**	**25**	**26**	**27**	**28**	**29**	**30**	**35**	**40**
Height (in.)						Weight (lb.)								
58	91	96	100	105	110	115	119	124	129	134	138	143	167	191
59	94	99	104	109	114	119	124	128	133	138	143	148	173	198
60	97	102	107	112	118	123	128	133	138	143	148	153	179	204
61	100	106	111	116	122	127	132	137	143	148	153	158	185	211
62	104	109	115	120	126	131	136	142	147	153	158	164	191	218
63	107	113	118	124	130	135	141	146	152	158	163	169	197	225
64	110	116	122	128	134	140	145	151	157	163	169	174	204	232
65	114	120	126	132	138	144	150	156	162	168	174	180	210	240
66	118	124	130	136	142	148	155	161	167	173	179	186	216	247
67	121	127	134	140	146	153	159	166	172	178	185	191	223	255
68	125	131	138	144	151	158	164	171	177	184	190	197	230	262
69	128	135	142	149	155	162	169	176	182	189	196	203	236	270
70	132	139	146	153	160	167	174	181	188	195	202	207	243	278
71	136	143	150	157	165	172	179	186	193	200	208	215	250	286
72	140	147	154	162	169	177	184	191	199	206	213	221	258	294
73	144	151	159	166	174	182	189	197	204	212	219	227	265	302
74	148	155	163	171	179	186	194	202	210	218	225	233	272	311
75	152	160	168	176	184	192	200	208	216	224	232	240	279	319
76	156	164	172	180	189	197	205	213	221	230	238	246	287	328

If your BMI is between 18.5 and 24.9, you are in the healthy BMI range. If it is equal to or over 25, you are considered overweight. If it is equal to or greater than 30, you are considered obese. (If it's below 18.5, you're too skinny and need to get some meat on those bones of yours!)

If a person has lots of muscle, he or she can be well into the 25–30 BMI range and not look overweight or be at risk for health issues related to being overweight. This is because the BMI doesn't take into account that muscle weighs more than fat.

Nutritionists often modify the BMI measurements to take into account different categories of weight and size. The numbers for men are slightly higher than for women.

Women Are:	
Underweight	If BMI is less than 19.1
Ideal weight	19.1 to 25.8
Marginally overweight	25.9 to 27.3
Overweight	27.4 to 32.2
Obese	32.3 to 44.8
Extremely obese	greater than 44.8

Men Are:	
Underweight	If BMI is less than 20.7
Ideal weight	20.7 to 26.4
Marginally overweight	26.5 to 27.8
Overweight	27.9 to 31.1
Obese	31.2 to 45.4
Extremely obese	greater than 45.4

Another measurement that professionals use is the waist/hip ratio. Measure your waist at its smallest place and your hips at their widest. Divide your waist measurement by your hip measurement. If the number is nearly 1.0 or greater, you are at greater risk for some health problems such as diabetes, heart disease, and certain kinds of cancer. For a healthy weight, a woman's ratio should be less than 0.80; a man's should be less than 0.95.

Your Attainable Goal

Yes, you can determine your target ideal size in many ways. We generally recommend that your primary goal should be based on a measurable size, such as jean size, dress size, or belt size. These are measures of how you actually look—to yourself and to others.

Although we are not fond of the bathroom scale, you can consider a weight-based measure if you're so inclined. But if those daily weight fluctuations (and you will have them) cause you to suffer emotional fluctuations, too, just stay off the scale and use the fit of your clothes as your guide.

Getting your body fat percentage into a healthy range is an admirable goal, too, but you might find only limited benefit from highly precise measurements. Body fat percentage is certainly not something you should measure with great frequency. With a regular routine of moderate strength exercises, you will *know* your body fat percentage is decreasing. You can see—and feel—the new muscle. That's a lot more fun.

With all that said, we strongly encourage you to create your ideal size goal or goals. They are not just destinations on a journey; they are your guideposts along the way. Think of them as friends, not as enemies. Embrace them with optimism and determination. In Chapters 25 and 26, we will show you powerful ways to win the mental game of weight loss. But for now, simply assume that you will reach your goals.

Here is a place to write down your goals. We recommend that you include your desired jean size and body fat percentage as two of your weight-loss measurements.

My Weight Loss Goals:

My desired jean size _____
My desired body fat percentage _____
My desired dress or belt size _____
My desired BMI _____
My desired weight _____
My preferred weight-loss goal is _____ using the _____ method

The Least You Need to Know

- ◆ Your ideal size is the one you want to be, the one that gives you the most energy, and the one that feels the best.

- ◆ All methods for determining your ideal size have advantages and drawbacks.

- ◆ Select your ideal size using a primary measure and focus on it.

- ◆ Affirm to yourself often that you are already at your ideal size.

Chapter 4

Stay the Course, Results Will Follow

In This Chapter

◆ Changing your attitudes about food

◆ Staying on your weight-loss program

◆ Right-sizing for you and your food

What do you have to show for all the time, energy, and money spent on weight loss in your life? Not much. In fact, you could be larger than ever before. If you aren't larger, perhaps you feel flabbier and more discouraged. You know your efforts haven't produced the desired results. What's not working?

A significant part of mastering your weight is conquering the barriers that get in your way. In this chapter, we tell you how to avoid and correct the common pitfalls you could encounter. These include weight-loss plateaus, discouragement, and using food to soothe stress and anxiety.

Staying the Course

A good weight-loss system is only as good as your commitment. With a balanced, practical system spiced with common sense, you can be successful. All systems are destined to fail, however, if you fail the system. An effective weight-loss system is one that incorporates the following aspects: how to eat, balanced nutrition, exercise, and attitude. Let's look at what you need to bring to a good weight-loss program for you to win at weight loss.

Tenacity and Patience

Tenacity is the most critical factor for weight loss. In the words of Winston Churchill, "Never, never, never, never, never give up."

Figure that it takes two to three months for a woman to lose a dress size healthfully. Ditto for a man to lose 2 inches of belt size. If you are starting at a size 20 and want to be a size 10, it could take as long as 15 months. Can you hang in there for the long haul?

You could be thinking to yourself, "Fifteen months! By then I'll be almost a year and a half older. Do I have to be larger than I want to be for 15 months?" You know the answer. It's yes. Think of it this way: you will be 15 months older anyway. When you get there, would you rather be overweight or your ideal size?

To reach your goal, don't allow yourself to be derailed by stress, depressed emotions, or an off-the-cuff comment from friends or family. Although you want quick results, it's easy to get discouraged when you don't see visible results right away. Weight loss takes as long as it takes.

Starting the Journey to Your Ideal Size

When you begin a weight-loss program, you are starting a growth process, just like planting a seed. After planting the seed, it needs time to germinate. If you become impatient to see the tiny green plant shoot and decide to dig up the seed to see whether it's germinating, you will kill the plant. Germination is the time for patience. As you eat nutritiously and exercise faithfully, you will see some changes, but you cannot reach your weight goal overnight, just as the seed doesn't sprout and produce beautiful flowers overnight.

Fruition is when the seed bears flowers and fruit. For you, the fruition of your goal is when those jeans fit comfortably. The attainment of your ideal size can take months and perhaps even years from when you begin. Be patient. Good things come to those who persevere and wait.

Thinspiration

Your body is your work of art, right? In the beginning, a painter's efforts are just oil and canvas. But eventually— voilà!—the painter creates a masterpiece. It will take time to turn your body into a master-piece, too. But you can do it!

Food, Food, Everywhere Food

We are bombarded with weight-loss advertising and news reports about the growing "size" of the population. At the same time, Madison Avenue tries to seduce us with advertising that promotes food and eating. The newsstand formula for selling check-out counter magazines is simple: picture a luscious-looking dessert and a headline that reads, "Lose 10 pounds in a week." These magazines fuel our national love-hate affair with food and eating.

Fast-food restaurants still tantalize us with offers to "supersize" our orders because of the extra "value" we get. Sit-down restaurants serve portions that are big enough for two or three people. We are repeatedly encouraged to assume that bigger is better ... even when it's not.

Supersized meals lead to supersized bodies. These hefty meals offer enough food to feed two, three, or four people. Rather than getting supersized meals, get a right-size meal. Get just enough to meet your body's needs and no more.

Today, food is more widely available and abundant for the average person than at any other time in the history of man, especially in first-world countries such as the United States. This hasn't always been the case. You don't have to go back far in history to find times when food was *not* plentiful. Many people lived in a feast-or-famine envi-ronment. When food was plentiful, they ate lots of it because they didn't know from where their next meal was coming. They ate richly whenever they could to store enough fat so that they could make it through the lean times. Today, in our country food is plentiful, but many people eat as their ancestors did—eagerly and anxiously— as though they don't know when they are going to eat again.

Practically any food you could possibly want is available right now within less than an hour's drive of your home. Even if you live away from a city, you can order your favorite foods through the Internet and mail-order catalogs. You can't even begin to eat all the food that is available to you.

Think of a T-shirt emblazoned with the saying "So much food, so little time." Hopefully that has not been your food motto. If it has, change it. How about a T-shirt that reads, "I eat all that I need but not more than I need." Or it might have a motto of "I eat plenty but not more than enough." These mottos add an elegance to eating that lets you be in control. It lets you transcend the caveman urge to fill up at every food station on your path through life.

For now, think about right-sizing both your body and your food intake. Plan to take in enough food to stay healthy and active. Plan to stop eating supersized meals before they supersize you.

Nothing Ventured, Nothing Lost

Have you almost given up on losing weight and getting to your ideal size? Has your weight-loss history led you to believe that being thin is only a temporary condition? Are you afraid to lose and gain yet one more time? If so, you are more normal than you might think.

Being afraid of failing at weight loss one more time can be immobilizing. Being immobilized by this fear is almost like giving up on yourself as a person, and you don't want to do that. You may be thinking, "So what's a couple of pounds or a couple more? It absolutely doesn't define who I am as a person. It doesn't speak to my value or my contributions." You are correct. However, it does speak to your interest in your health and your sense of self-esteem. The healthier you are, the more you can contribute to yourself and others for many more years.

By using the advice in this book, you can be assured that you're doing what is necessary to give you the benefits you want. You will show yourself and others your courage and interest in being around for the long haul.

Reaching Plateaus

As you lose weight, you might hit a plateau. Your best efforts seem to stall. You stay the same size regardless of what you do. One client, Deborah, went from a size 26 to a size 18 very quickly, within six months. Then she stayed at a size 18 for almost a year before her weight started down again. Deborah had the wisdom to wait it out. She kept to her eating and exercise plans and continued to live normally. Eventually, her body began to release more excess fat and today she is delighted to be a size 14.

What happens during plateaus? We like to think of them as "still points." Let's compare a plateau in weight loss to water boiling. You put the water into a pot on the stove and turn the heat on high. Not much happens for what seems like a long time (especially if you are watching the pot boil!). During that time, thermal energy is transferred from the burner into the water. As the thermal energy is transferred, the water increases in temperature until it reaches the boiling point. The thermal energy is finally converted into kinetic energy, and you can observe the pot boil.

So it is with weight loss. At the time when nothing seems to be happening, plenty is going on in your body that can't be seen. The body must change a lot as it loses weight. As the body converts fat into energy, the liver detoxifies the by-products and releases them to be excreted as waste products. The body reshapes itself, using up plenty of vitamins, minerals, and trace elements as it does so. The body works extra hard as it releases fat. You should expect that it would rest and regroup from time to time.

Emotionally, plateaus are challenging. You want results and want them fast. Deborah's patience and tenacity pulled her through a year-long plateau. A plateau is the time to stay the course, say aloud your weight-loss affirmations, refine your nutritional and exercise programs, and keep the faith.

Food Is Only Food

Food is excellent for supplying nutrition, energy, and sensory delights, but it does not have magical powers. It can't heal a broken heart. It can't make a skinned knee stop hurting.

People turn to food to do the impossible—to make emotional pain go away, to avoid loneliness, and to improve high-anxiety moments. People want food to solve some basic issues of life. It can't. It has no power. You have the power to do those things.

If you have ever hoped that food would solve things, just remember how disappointed you were when the food failed you. Perhaps you have returned to food again and again, seeing whether things have changed and that somehow food could solve anything.

Thinspiration

Overeating is never the solution, no matter what the problem. It only leads to more problems. Overeating can't heal a broken heart, make you more comfortable at a party, or eliminate stress. All that it can do is add on more pounds.

By now, you absolutely know it can't. But are you still hoping? This kind of hope is terrifically fattening. Give it up. Find wiser ways to solve life's problems.

Food is also not the same as love. Certainly, we prepare food for our families because we love them, but whether they eat the food has nothing to do with whether they are accepting of our love. Ditto for someone preparing food for you. You are not required to eat everything just because someone made it for you. Show your love in many other ways and let food be just food.

Guilt Is a Choice, Not a Requirement

Ever notice how guilt about overeating begets more overeating? Take a binger who is usually overly careful about her food intake. She counts calories or fat grams (or both) and can be seen obsessing over whether to have dressing on her chef salad at lunch.

Every once in a while, though, that strong and virtually undeniable urge to overeat surfaces, and she gives in. At those times, she forgets about calories and fat grams. She eats heavy foods, laden with all the richness she has been denying herself. At first it feels good, but then it feels awful. Not only is her stomach stuffed and extended, all her careful eating has been ruined. She feels horrible and hates her behavior and herself. She can't understand why she did it. Remorse builds up inside her. The tears come after this seemingly crazy behavior.

So does guilt. This feeling starts eating at her. How could she? What's wrong with her? Bingeing is a bad thing to do. How can she ever atone for this mistake? The guilt wells up inside. Soon she is eating to assuage the guilt. The guilt is layered just like that magnificent torte she inhaled. Guilt for what she did, guilt for ruining her diet, guilt at such bizarre behavior, guilt at being overweight. Talk about the guilt of the world resting on someone's shoulders.

The more she binges and the more she overeats, the guiltier she feels. Then she eats more to deal with the yucky feelings. Cause and effect become blurred. What is a person to do?

The first step in breaking the guilt-eating syndrome is to forgive oneself. Forgive yourself for all the offenses you thought you did: overeating, bingeing, being fat, being out of control, you name it. As you do this, the guilt releases, and you are free and fresh. Then wait until you are hungry and eat normally until your body's hunger is satisfied.

Guilt is a useless, unproductive emotion when it comes to reaching your ideal size. Tell yourself, "It is okay and important to eat. I eat just enough food and not more than my body needs." You'll discover that eating without guilt is a great feeling, one you will enjoy regularly as you gain mastery over your eating habits. Guilt ruins almost all dieting attempts.

> **Body of Knowledge**
>
> In any situation in which you have overeaten, forgive yourself. You simply forgot that you were at your ideal size and that you have mastered your weight and eating. Then wait until you are hungry and eat enough but not too much.

Lucy's Losing Journey

I, Lucy, was a classic yo-yo dieter in college and through my early 30s. I tried many diets and food schemes such as vegetarian macrobiotic eating. I lost weight many times but always regained it. My top weight was 175 or a large size 14. As a heavy-duty binger obsessed with eating and food, I thought I was addicted to sugar and chocolate.

I cried a lot about my weight, and even worse, I never stopped thinking about food and eating. By the time I was finally ready to release my weight issue forever, I most wanted to lose my constant mental obsessing about food and my weight.

By then, having spent a small fortune trying every popular weight-loss program, I began looking for alternative methods. Over a year or two, I read a couple of books, went to several counselors and classes, and finally figured it out. I realized that I could walk away from my weight issue and never return. It was a choice I made.

By using affirmations and visualizations (which are discussed in Chapter 25), I stopped overeating and began to eat normal foods. I forgave myself for all the pain I was causing my loved ones and myself. Within six months I was wearing a size 6, and I have stayed there for more than 20 years. I have no idea what I weigh because I don't use scales. My jeans fit. I enjoy food. I eat some sugar and chocolate in moderation along with a nutritionally balanced diet. I seldom eat starches.

I easily maintain my size 6 by doing the same things I did to lose my weight—eating normally, that is, eating only when I was hungry and stopping when I had eaten enough food, before I was full. I exercise about five to six hours a week, doing the Five Tibetans (see Part 4) and cardio exercises daily, plus two Pilates sessions a week. For recreation, my husband and I go hiking.

The Least You Need to Know

- Should you reach a weight-loss plateau, keep on keeping on and doing what works.

- With the vast abundance of food available in the United States, there is no need for you to overeat at any meal.

- Food is not love and can't solve life's problems.

- Guilt is useless and counterproductive when it comes to weight loss.

Part 2

Your Basic Weight-Loss Program

You body is an amazing machine. So amazing, in fact, that it instinctively knows how, when, and what to eat to lose weight and keep it off. The only problem is that it's easy to override your body's inner wisdom. In this part of the book, you learn how to once again listen to your body's subtle signals of hunger and satiation. But that's not all—you'll learn how to work with your body to naturally boost your metabolism so that you can actually eat more food and still lose weight. And you'll find it much easier to keep the weight off.

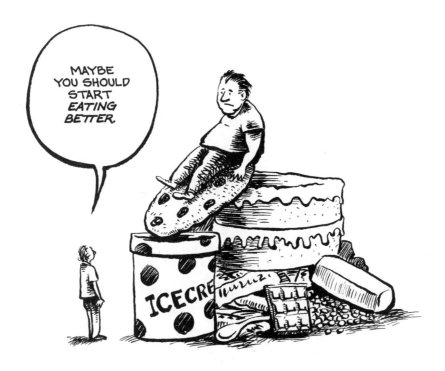

Chapter 5

Eating Based on Your Body's Needs

In This Chapter

- ◆ Eating as your body and stomach direct
- ◆ Eliminating poor eating habits
- ◆ Hearing your body's hunger signals
- ◆ Eating 0–5 using a hunger scale

The body is utterly amazing. It takes food in and processes it into energy while extracting nutrients. It manages to excrete what it doesn't need and to store any excess energy supplies as fat. Aaah, there's the rub. Your body's fat-storage system is a natural part of the body's digestive process. It's programmed to add layers of fat, especially when it gets more food than it needs! Now your task is to use up those fat stores and avoid storing even more fat.

If Only Your Body Could Talk

An essential part of losing weight and keeping it off is learning how to listen to your body. We all wish it could just say what it wants. Although your body doesn't have an oral language, it does communicate. Certainly, you know when your body hurts because you feel pain. You know when it needs rest because you get the unmistakable cues of nodding off, yawns, and sleepiness. But are you able to clearly hear your body communicate when it is time for you to eat and when it is time to stop eating?

Infants know these signals well. So do animals that live in the wilderness. Most adult humans don't remember the language of hunger and satiation. Infants cry to signal that they need a feeding. Infants know how they are doing by how they feel. If they feel good, everything is fine in their world. If they don't feel good, if something hurts or irritates them, they let mama know right away. By observing an infant cry for food, you can tell that hunger is an actual discomfort. It is felt in the stomach.

Infants also seem to know instinctively when to stop eating. You can tell when they have had enough milk because they simply stop feeding. Mid-bottle, mid-drop, it doesn't matter to an infant how much milk is left. Mama may want the infant to drink more milk so that the infant sleeps through the night, but the infant refuses. Why? Because he or she instinctively knows that even one more drop may produce feelings of discomfort—of being too full and even stuffed. That discomfort is so significant that an infant will not risk the irritation. Besides, he or she is already satisfied.

"Full" Is Not Your Friend

Changing your perception about being *full* is the critical first step toward reaching your ideal size. Notice that an infant does not keep feeding on milk until he or she is full.

Lean Lingo

The feeling of a **full** stomach is a signal that you have eaten too much food. Typically, people who are overweight are accustomed to eating until they are full. Usually this means eating a quantity of food bigger than their own fist—give or take.

Full is actually an uncomfortable feeling. Wanting to get full from eating is an urge that develops later in life due to social pressure and outside messages from family and peers. Infants feed only until they have enough nourishment but not too much. They eat until the hunger urges abate or until their hunger is satisfied and the stomach is comfortable.

The good news is that you were once an infant and you knew how to listen to your body's hunger signals. You have since changed your eating habits to accommodate social norms and emotions, but at the beginning of your life, you ate based on your body's needs. Let's learn how to get closer to those original instincts about food. You may never need to feel full again … and you will be thrilled with the results. You'll be losing weight and attaining your ideal size.

Hunger Is Your Friend

Hunger is good. Hunger is a natural part of your body, and it would be disastrous not to feel hunger. Without the capability to feel hunger, a wild animal would die from starvation. Hunger is a grand thing because it tells us when it's time to eat. Every time you feel true hunger in your stomach, it's time to eat. For some of us, that's three times a day. For some, it could be six times a day. For some, the frequency of feeling hunger pangs varies from day to day.

It's never wise to do things to avoid feeling hunger. You are supposed to feel hunger so that you can know when it's time to eat because eating helps sustain life. You may be thinking that your hunger is out of control. Most often, it isn't out of control; rather, you have either denied or ignored your true hunger feelings for so long that you don't recognize them. You can trust real stomach hunger.

However, there's a sort of fake hunger. It comes from stress and anxiety or other emotions, sometimes from appetite stimulants such as alcohol, prescription drugs, illegal drugs, or a lack of sleep. The fake hunger is just that. The communication doesn't come from a hunger pang; more likely it comes from the mouth, as in an oral chewing need, from emotional feelings, or from thirst.

Feeling true hunger pangs and understanding how your body communicates hunger are important tools. They make a big difference in your overall success, regardless of which eating program you use.

> **Body of Knowledge**
>
> Stomach muscle contractions cause stomach growls. When food is in the stomach, the muscles move food through into the small intestine. When your stomach is empty, however, you can hear and feel the "growls." Usually, this is a signal that you are hungry, and it's time to eat.

How to Feel Hunger

Hunger is a pain, and it is felt somewhere above, below, or behind your belly button. Hunger feels different for different people. For some, it is almost like a muscle contraction. For others, it's an empty or void feeling.

To become acquainted with your hunger, wait to eat until you feel a hunger pang. For most people, it takes about two to five hours after the previous meal to feel hunger.

Pay close attention to your stomach initially to feel hunger. Identify where the physical feelings are located. Listen intently to any rumbling or growling. Perhaps you are chuckling at the thought of "listening" to your stomach, but learning your own body signals is remarkably powerful.

What Gets in the Way

Listening to your hunger is incredibly useful in getting to your ideal size. Unfortunately, many of us have a tough time getting the message because certain conditions block us from "hearing" them. Here are a few of the common blockages:

Low blood sugar. If you miss feeling the hunger pang and instead become light-headed, jittery, irritable, or cranky, go ahead and eat. You could have low blood sugar, which speaks more loudly than hunger pangs, at least at first. When you eat based on the nutritional advice in Part 3—by getting protein, fats, and carbohydrates at every meal—your low blood sugar will lessen, and you can feel your hunger pangs better.

Painkillers. If you are on painkillers, either prescription or over-the-counter, you might not be able to feel the sensations of hunger. Other medications, such as anti-seizure or anti-convulsant medications, can also block hunger feelings. If this is your situation, be sure to read the section "A Fist Full of Food" later in this chapter.

Nervous stomach. If you feel anxiety as pain in your stomach, you might mistake the anxiety pain for a hunger pang. If this happens to you, see the section "A Fist Full of Food" later in this chapter.

Too busy to feel. If you get so busy that you can shut out the world, most likely you can also shut out hunger feelings. Set your watch or alarm to ring every hour to remind you to ask your stomach whether it's time to eat (that is, if it's hungry).

No experience. Perhaps you have ignored your body's hunger communications for most of your life. You may not be able to feel them because you are out of practice. Some people, in fact, never let themselves get hungry. If this is your situation, take time to listen and hear your body's faint and subtle hunger messages. The more you are able to take the time to listen, the louder the messages become. Eventually, you will hear them talking to you loud and clear.

Smile when you feel stomach hunger. It is confirming that you haven't been overfeeding yourself. And good news, when you feel stomach hunger, it's time to eat. Then eat just the right amount of food to feel comfortable and not full.

Satisfaction

As previously mentioned, an infant stops feeding when his or her hunger is satisfied. How does the baby know? The answer is similar to the fable of Goldilocks and the three bears. Goldilocks looked for the porridge, the chair, and the bed that felt just right. The same should be true with your stomach and feeling satisfied. The satisfied stomach isn't a little bit hungry or a little bit full. It feels just right.

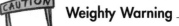

Weighty Warning

In our culture, when children want to be excused from the dinner table, we often ask, "Are you full?" Change this now to "Did you get enough?" Don't encourage eating until full, but only to the point of satisfaction.

Being satisfied is pretty much a nonfeeling. You aren't full, but your stomach hunger pangs have ceased. You have room to take a deep breath. The waistband on your pants doesn't cut into the flesh of your waist. You have enough energy to take a walk or do an activity. You don't feel full, just satisfied.

What Do You Prefer: Full or Satisfied?

Answer the following questions:

1. Do you usually go back for seconds at dinner or lunch?
   ☐ Yes ☐ No

2. Do you "supersize" your meal at fast-food restaurants?
   ☐ Yes ☐ No

3. Do you loosen your belt or change to looser clothes at the end of a meal more than once a month?
   ☐ Yes ☐ No

4. Do you eat a dessert at the end of a meal even when you're satisfied and have had plenty of food?
   ☐ Yes ☐ No

5. Do you regularly drink more than one beer or glass of wine with a meal?
   ☐ Yes ☐ No

6. Do you usually eat everything on your plate, as in being a member of The Clean Plate Club?
   ☐ Yes ☐ No

7. After dinner, do you usually sit and watch TV or do another sedentary activity?
   ☐ Yes ☐ No

8. Do you eat more than one piece of bread along with everything else on your plate at a main meal?
   ☐ Yes ☐ No

9. Do you binge eat, or eat to satisfy emotional hunger?
   ☐ Yes ☐ No

10. Do you continue to snack or eat throughout the evening?
    ☐ Yes ☐ No

If you answered "Yes" to more than one or two of these questions, you probably have a habit of eating until you're full or stuffed. As you work toward reaching your ideal size, you'll adopt new habits that let you answer "No" to these questions.

Two Simple Rules for Eating Naturally

Eating naturally is eating based on honoring your body's hunger communications. Take a cue from infants who eat only when they are hungry. You need to remember only two broad rules: 1) only eat when you feel a hunger pang; 2) only eat enough food to get satisfied, not enough to get full.

Virtually any healthy eating plan or diet program you choose will work if you honor these two key body communications. If you don't honor them, frankly, you should expect to fail.

A Fist Full of Food

Make a fist and observe the size of it. This is about the size of your stomach. Oh dear, you may be thinking, "How did all of that food I ate last night fit into a space so small?" Good question. First, realize that you almost certainly ate more than you needed to feel satisfied. Next, understand that your stomach is a muscle that can expand to accommodate a great amount of food. Just ask anyone who is a binge eater.

Usually, eating an amount of food the size of your fist is enough to feel satisfied … give or take, based on the day, the weather, the cycles of the moon, and other unspecified mysteries of life and eating! To figure out the amount of food to eat based on comparing it to the size of your fist, you've got to imagine the food after you've chewed it. Oh, ick, you may think. Imagine that the air is taken out of such foods as a salad.

Seriously, you can't go wrong eating an amount of food the size of your fist three or four times a day. You certainly won't gain weight. Better yet, you'll start releasing stored fat.

Eating Less Means More Satisfaction

You may be studying the size of your fist right now, already feeling deprived. "That's not much food for me," you think. You're right, that's not much food, yet it is plenty of food to support your body. A fistful is still plenty of food to sustain your life, give you energy, release excess fat stores, look great, feel great, and get healthier.

Make sure that you eat the most absolutely delicious and nutritious foods and your favorite foods first; otherwise, you won't have room for them. This applies to buffets, eating out, and parties—every time you are hungry. Be sure to eat slowly so you savor every morsel of food you eat. The taste and sensuous pleasure of the food last longer that way.

Going Against Your Body's Natural Flow

When you overeat, you upset your body's designed eating rhythms. Ideally, you only eat when hungry, you stop eating when you have enough, and you let your body digest that food before you have more. Being overweight means eating against your body's best interests.

Overweight people eat in several ways that are counterproductive. All of these ways of eating (described in the sections that follow) are harmful to the body's digestive system and to health. All of them basically ignore the body's hunger signals.

The Continual Feeder

This person always seems to be eating something. The continual eater never gives the body a beginning or ending to a meal. The stomach of a continual feeder never gets to rest. Think of watching TV on the sofa with a bag of potato chips. All of a sudden, it seems, the potato chips are gone, and the person can't remember eating them. Continual feeders often dislike the feelings of hunger. So they avoid hunger feelings by continually feeding.

The Big-Meal Fan

This person wants lots of food at every meal. Somehow he or she doesn't feel complete unless the stomach is stuffed with food. The big-meal person can sometimes consume up to six fistfuls of food at every meal. The big-meal eater usually prefers bulk to quality. This person likes supersized meals and thinks that all-you-can-eat buffets are a great value. Big-meal eaters think that a hunger pang is the cue to "order big and eat big."

The Binge Eater

Every couple of days or weeks, this person binges on food, any kind of food. Of course, binge eaters often have favorite food indulgences, foods they prefer for binges. Usually the binge eater eats to excess when alone, but you might find this person stuffing in food at a cocktail party or social event.

The binge eater goes on automatic pilot and almost unconsciously (usually at night) eats and eats and eats until just below the bursting point. He or she doesn't burst, but the body's sensitive and gentle communication system gets abused. A large amount of food makes the digestive system work extra hard. It not only has to digest all that food; it has to store it as fat.

Take heart. If any of these describe your habits, remember that you are not alone, nor "incurable." As you learn to listen to and honor your body's hunger communications, you will eliminate the unproductive habits that hurt you and destroy your weight-loss efforts.

> **Thinspiration**
>
> The binge eater often uses eating to compensate for other problems in life. It's helpful to address those problems directly by using self-help techniques such as journaling or by working with a professional counselor or by finding a suitable substitute, like knitting or exercising.

> **Lean Lingo**
>
> A **hunger scale** is a numeric system designed to help you "score" the hunger levels of your stomach at any time.

The 0–5 Hunger Scale

Using a personal *hunger scale* is so fundamental to weight management that you will wonder why you haven't used one until now. Here's how one works.

The hunger scale helps you rate your hunger on a scale of 0–10. Here are the key reference numbers to understand:

Hunger Number	What It Means
0	*Empty:* The hunger point at which an infant cries or an adult has a hunger pang. When you're at 0, it's time to eat.
5	*Satisfied or comfortable:* When an infant stops feeding or when an adult feels a neutral feeling, neither hungry nor full. When it's time to stop eating.
7	*Full:* When you feel pressure inside the stomach from overeating. This is fattening.
10	*Stuffed:* When you feel as though you are can't-eat-another-bite stuffed and are highly uncomfortable from eating way too much food. This is highly fattening.

Using a hunger scale gives you excellent feedback about your eating habits. It can have a profound impact on your weight-loss efforts immediately.

What's Your Number?

On a scale of 0 to 10—with 0 being empty, 5 being comfortable, 7 being full, and 10 being stuffed, what is your hunger number right now? Close your eyes and focus your attention on your stomach, which is somewhere around your navel. Set aside any analytical or intellectual data you have about when you last ate and simply let your stomach give you a number. By the way, when you hear its number, thank your stomach for the information.

What does your number mean? If it's 0, it's time to eat. If it is above 0, wait until your stomach registers 0 before you eat.

Toward the end of a meal—and definitely before you have second helpings—stop and ask your stomach what its hunger number is. If it's 5, stop eating. If it's 4, you have room for some more food. If it's 6 or above, stop eating and forgive yourself for having overeaten. Wait until you are at 0 before you eat again.

It's possible to get below 0. This happens if you ignore your hunger signals, skip meals, or have low blood sugar. You can also get below 0 if for some reason you can't eat when you're hungry. Such reasons could be that food isn't available, you're in a business meeting, or so on. You could feel lightheaded, jittery, irritable, or headachy. The urge at that time is to "eat everything now." Don't do that. Instead, here is what to do if you get below 0:

◆ Eat a little something to get up to 0. This could be a piece of fruit, a cracker, juice, or some other food.

◆ Wait 10 to 15 minutes until your stomach hunger level is at 0.

◆ Eat normally, up to or below 5.

The beauty of this system is its simplicity. After you try this a handful of times, you'll be amazed at what you learn about your eating habits.

Snacking for Weight Loss

Let's say you're planning to eat dinner at 7 P.M., but it's only 5 P.M., and your stomach is already empty and announcing its hunger. You are at 0. This is a great time for a snack. You can eat a little something to get your hunger number up to 2 or 3 to tide you over until dinner. It wouldn't make much sense to eat up to 5 because then you wouldn't be hungry when dinner is served.

Snacks are great for whenever you are at 0 but it isn't mealtime. You can take snacks with you just in case you get to 0 when no one else with you is hungry. That way, you don't get overly hungry and famished. Overly hungry means you could eat the proverbial house. A little snack here and there prevents inhaling your food at the next meal.

Only eat snacks when you need them, that is when you are at 0 and it isn't time for a regular meal. Some people need snacks daily; some don't.

The Least You Need to Know

◆ Your body instinctively knows when to eat and when to stop eating.

◆ Only eat when your stomach is hungry, that is, at a 0. Stop eating when you have had enough food but before you are full, at a 5.

◆ The size of your unstretched stomach is about the size of your fist.

◆ Snacks are a great way to honor your body's hunger signals.

Chapter 6

Starve Your Body, Gain Weight

In This Chapter

- ◆ How a caveman's biology affects your weight loss
- ◆ Avoiding starvation metabolism
- ◆ Taking advantage of your powerful biological eating force
- ◆ Boosting your metabolism

Have you ever wondered why you gained your weight back after successfully losing it? You don't lack willpower or self-discipline. Instead, you are the victim of your own biology. Your biology makes you regain weight just as fast as you originally took it off. To keep weight off, you need to learn how your biology works and how to work with it to get to your ideal size and stay there.

You will learn how many of the popular diet recommendations can actually make you gain weight in the long term and make it more difficult to lose weight after that. You will learn how to avoid yo-yo dieting and the flabbier body that goes with it.

The Caveman and You

Your body is utterly amazing. From the food it consumes, it derives energy and nutrients. What your body doesn't need for energy immediately, it stores as fat for later use.

The good news, biologically speaking, is that your stores of fat are great protection against an upcoming famine. Like most mammals, humans with a good layer of fat on their bodies can live for several weeks without eating. You may get restless when you haven't eaten in a few hours, but the truth is that you could live quite a while before your next meal. You would eventually feel weak and lethargic, but you could still survive.

So hooray for fat, your protection against famine! But what happens when that famine never comes? As long as you keep eating more than your body needs for fuel, the body keeps storing more fat. Today in the United States, most of us don't need to concern ourselves with the fear of not having enough food, but our biology is still quite primitive. It is very close to that of our ancient ancestors, the caveman and cavewoman. Our present-day genome, the basic human genetic code, is almost identical to that of humans who lived 40,000 years ago. Yes, we rely on cell phones and computers, automobiles and airplanes, but biologically we aren't much different from the hunter-gatherers who lived during the Stone Age.

The caveman lived between the extremes of feast and famine. When he was fortunate enough to kill a large mammal, his whole family—perhaps even the whole tribe—feasted on the delicious meat. It provided high-quality protein, fats, B vitamins, and trace minerals that they needed for survival. Meat provided these in bio-accessible concentrations better than any other single food source. At other times, the lean times, the caveman ate berries, fish, and plants until he once again found more game.

During times of famine, the caveman's *metabolism* would slow down to conserve energy. When possible, his body would increase his fat stores by taking even the meager amount of food he did eat and storing it as fat. Why fat? Because fat is a more efficient fuel than muscle. The more fat that was stored, the longer the caveman could survive during a famine.

When he and the other members of the tribe feasted on the game meat, they were enjoying excess and abundant food. The caveman's body was clever. It knew that there could be a famine in the future, so it planned for contingencies. Any excess food eaten was stored as fat to prepare for the famine to come. The body handled the natural swings of feast and famine in elegant ways that ensured the survival of the species. Yes, too bad we don't think of these ways as elegant today!

Your biology is designed to do exactly what the caveman's did. Your body will conserve energy and store fat when it senses that it isn't getting enough food and nourishment, and your body stores fat when you overeat. Does this sound as though you are in a double bind? You add body fat if you undereat, and you add body fat if you overeat.

The solution to the dilemma is fundamentally simple: get enough food on a day-to-day basis for energy and nutrition, but not more than enough and not less than enough.

Lean Lingo _____

The general term **metabolism** refers to all the changes occurring in digested foodstuffs in the body from their absorption until their elimination. Your basal metabolism rate is the rate of energy metabolism required to keep the body alive. As you increase your metabolic rate, getting to your ideal size is easier.

Your Body Is an Engine

Your body acts like an engine that is constantly in operation. Food is its fuel. It burns the fuel to keep going. But your body's engine actually consists of millions of living cells, which are themselves tiny engines. Each cell in your body requires energy to stay alive. Food provides the energy.

Your body derives the energy and nutrients it needs from foods. Your body is a marvelous engine that keeps you alive by converting food into energy through a vast number of chemical processes.

Your metabolic rate measures the rate at which your individual body is using up energy (as measured in _calories_) to stay alive. It's not a rate that remains constantly the same. Your metabolic rate varies throughout the day and throughout your life, depending on your level of activity and other factors.

Lean Lingo _____

A **calorie** of food refers to the amount of energy available to the body from the oxidation or digestion of food. When used as a calorie of food, it means that when a food is oxidized in the tissues of the body, it releases 1,000 times that amount of energy to be used by the body.

Your basal metabolic rate (BMR) describes the rate at which your body uses energy (also measured in calories) in a totally relaxed mode. It is usually measured in the morning after a comfortable night's rest, when you are relaxed in bed, before breakfast. (Sounds nice, doesn't it?!)

A Closer Look at Metabolic Rate

John, a 28-year-old mechanic whose hobby is mountain biking, claims to have a "high metabolism." He probably believes that his basal metabolic rate is higher than the norm. He may be right. We don't all have the same BMR. The following are known to influence basal metabolic rate:

- **Age.** The BMR gradually decreases with age due to inactivity and lower muscle mass.

- **Sex.** The BMR is generally a little lower in women than in men.

- **Sleep.** Inadequate sleep over time will decrease your BMR.

- **Exercise.** Systematic exercise will increase your BMR.

- **Nourishment.** Prolonged undernourishment will decrease your BMR.

- **Thyroid hormone.** Poor thyroid functioning decreases your BMR.

- **Stress Levels**. High stress levels reduce your BMR.

- **Dehydration**. Inadequate water intake decreases your BMR.

- **Body fat percentage**. A high body fat percentage decreases your BMR; a low body fat percentage increases it.

John, because he's young, muscular, and athletic, probably does have a higher basal metabolic rate than Jim, a middle-aged accountant who struggles to push the lawn mower on Saturdays. John's higher BMR will help him burn calories faster than Jim does … even when he's asleep. His engine is idling more quickly; it uses up fuel more quickly.

But John may have been referring to the fact that he burns through a lot more calories every week because his overall metabolism operates at a higher level. The physical activities he engages in, both at work and in leisure, burn calories more quickly than sedentary activities. His engine is working harder; it uses up fuel more quickly.

The rate at which you burn calories is lowest while you sleep and greatest when you physically work hard. Here's a guide that describes the approximate calories burned during various types of work. Keep in mind that these "burn rates" will vary from person to person, so use this as a guide to the relative energy used up for each level of activity.

Activity	Calories per Hour
Sleeping	65
Very light work or sitting at rest	100
Light work	120
Moderate work	175
Heavy-duty work	375

As you can see, energy stored in the body is metabolized much more quickly when physical exertion increases. So let's compare the calories burned in a typical day by John and Jim.

John	Calories
8 hrs of sleep at 65 cal/hr	520
8 hrs of work as a mechanic at 175 cal/hr	1,400
4 hrs of everyday light activity at 120 cal/hr	480
2 hrs of mountain biking at 375 cal/hr	750
2 hrs of eating, TV, and so on at 100 cal/hr	200
Subtotal	*3,350*
Calories burned during digestion	335
Total requirement for 24 hours	3,685
Jim	**Calories**
8 hrs of sleep at 65 cal/hr	520
8 hrs of work at a desk job at 120 cal/hr	960
4 hrs of everyday light activities at 120 cal/hr	480
4 hrs of eating, TV, and so on at 100 cal/hr	400
Subtotal	*2,360*
Calories burned during digestion	189
Total requirement for 24 hours	2,549

Without even considering that John probably has a higher basal metabolic rate because of his regular physical activity, you can see the dramatic difference in caloric requirements because of the lifestyle differences between John and Jim. John can eat 1,100 more calories in a day than Jim without gaining weight.

Starvation Metabolism

Our ancestors, the caveman and woman, faced daily hardships that meant they couldn't always count on where their next meals were coming from. During lean eating times, their bodies automatically went into starvation metabolism. So can yours. This is not good.

Starvation metabolism refers to a slowing of the basal metabolic rate brought on when the body is undernourished. The body, instinctively fearing starvation, naturally burns calories more slowly to survive longer. It also hoards energy, builds up fat stores, and causes the yo-yo dieting syndrome.

> **CAUTION**
>
> **Weighty Warning**
>
> Going on a strict diet to lose just enough weight for a class reunion, wedding, or special party is ultimately fattening because your body shifts into starvation metabolism and makes up for lost time after the big event.

It's a cruel joke that our bodies will kick into starvation metabolism at the most inopportune time. We're not starving. We're just trying to lose weight! Most people who slip into starvation metabolism do so when they go on a highly restricted diet for a couple of weeks or a couple of months. Few people can sustain this kind of diet for long. Then, when the diet is abandoned, the dieter starts making up for lost time. The maintenance plan goes right out the door and in come the cookies, cakes, pastries, and candy. Adding insult to injury, the body then swings into excess mode and starts storing fat in anticipation of another perceived famine. Unfortunately, we willingly prolong the vicious cycle by again starting a highly restrictive diet.

The solution to this modern form of feast or famine is to eat balanced and nutritious foods in a weight-loss system that includes exercise, good eating habits, and positive thin thoughts. The system needs to be gentle, forgiving, and healthy so that a person can stay on the system over a lifetime, not just for a quickie weight loss.

Suppose that you have already given up restrictive diets and have sworn off the ensuing compensatory food flings. You could still be putting yourself into starvation metabolism, perhaps on a day-to-day basis. Here's how you could be doing this and the corrections to make.

When you get a hunger signal from your stomach that you are now at 0 and it is time to eat, be sure you eat within an hour or so. Do not skip this meal. If you do, your body will get the message that food is not available and that it must start hoarding energy. It begins to store fat. If it's time to eat and you are not hungry—that is, if your stomach is not at 0—you can miss a meal and not go into starvation metabolism. If you are hungry, however, be sure to eat.

Monday morning is often diet morning. Sally, who repeatedly struggles with her weight issue, decides that this Monday is the perfect time to start a new diet. So how does she begin? She skips breakfast. Think of all the calories saved right off the bat, she thinks to herself. She also limits herself to some kind of light food for lunch, maybe even skips that meal, too. Sally is feeling quite proud of her willpower and self-discipline.

But come late afternoon when Sally arrives home from work, something inside her cannot stand it any longer. She might feel depressed, fatigued, and/or discouraged. She starts to eat, and by bedtime has eaten enough food for three or four meals, getting more food than she needs. Overall she ate more food for the day than she eats normally. By evening, she was feasting. What happened?

By skipping a good breakfast and lunch, Sally put herself into starvation metabolism. The body started storing fat and slowed metabolism to conserve energy. By late in the day, Sally was "starving," so to speak, and her biology insisted that she eat. And eat our dieter did … to make up for the skipped meals. Within one day's time, the body had slowed metabolism, begun storing fat because the dieter was acting like she was in a famine, and later stored fat because the dieter was feasting.

For many people, the same scenario plays itself out day after day, and they are at a loss for why they are gaining weight. Even if dieters eat the same amount of calories in a day of feast and famine as they do on a normal day when they eat three meals plus snacks, feast-and-famine eating makes them gain weight.

The very best way to avoid slipping into starvation metabolism is to eat when your body is hungry. Skip meals only if your hunger level, as measured on the 0–10 scale, is above 0 (that is, it's 1, 2, 3, or higher).

Eat for Optimum Energy and Metabolism

Your body likes balanced meals. When you favor one kind of nutrient over another, the body's metabolism can slow down. Judy was a 48-year-old woman who worked out at the gym doing cardio and weight training five to six mornings a week for at least 45 minutes. She was gaining weight. She insisted that she was not overeating.

We tested her metabolic rate and found that her metabolism was very slow and sluggish. She was confused. Wasn't exercise supposed to boost her metabolism?

We reviewed her eating over the previous couple of days. She had eaten no fat, no meat, and only soy shakes for meals. Her food intake had been like this for months. She wasn't getting enough calories, and her diet was out of balance. She was in starvation metabolism. Without enough fat and high-quality protein, the body acts like it is starving. Judy needed to add to her diet some essential fatty acids; complete, high-quality protein such as meat, eggs, or real cheese; and plenty more vegetables and fruits. Only then did her exercise regime jump-start her metabolism and let her lose weight.

If you are not eating enough proteins, fats, or fruits and vegetables and are instead filling up on breads and starches, you could be in starvation metabolism. If you are centering meals around pasta and starches such as bread, wheat, rice, white potatoes, and corn, you could also be compromising your metabolic rate.

Gimme a Cup o' Joe

Oh, how we love our coffee and other caffeine-laden drinks! Unfortunately, they can be the enticing culprits that lead you into starvation metabolism. Let's say you have that first cup of coffee in the morning just after you awaken. It gives you zip and energy. It wakes you up. So far, so good. It can also keep you from getting hungry for breakfast. Not so good.

Caffeine inhibits your ability to feel hunger. In other words, it gives you a false negative for hunger. So you most likely skip breakfast. Come midmorning, you want a little something to eat because your blood sugar has crashed. This is due to not eating and also because of the lift and drop caused by caffeine. If food is inconvenient at the moment, you may just settle on another caffeinated beverage.

You actually might be using caffeine as a way to not have to eat. Well, it works for that, but you are getting into starvation metabolism because you aren't eating regularly.

Body of Knowledge

Be sure to check the label on your favorite soft drinks and pain medications. Caffeine is contained in most dark-colored sodas such as Coke and Pepsi and is also in Mountain Dew and Orange Fanta.

Recent studies have shown that drinking two to three cups of coffee per day can elevate cortisol levels. Cortisol is an adrenal hormone that adds weight around the waist and tummy.

Caffeine is in coffee and tea, both black and green. It's an ingredient in many soft drinks and diet soft drinks, appetite suppressants, and over-the-counter painkillers, diet pills, and supplements. Caffeine is also in kola nut and guarana.

We know you love your coffee and caffeine, and the good news is that you most likely do not need to give it up. But you might need to change the way you use it. Rather than having your coffee or caffeine before a meal, have it with your meal and have only a cup or two in your day. That's right, have your cup of joe *with* breakfast, not before breakfast. The same goes for any caffeine you have throughout the day—have it with food. That way, you avoid starvation metabolism and can still enjoy a cup of joe.

Thinspiration

Breakfast is such an important meal that we encourage you to eat it even if you're not feeling hungry. This is the only time we recommend that you break the rule to eat 0–5. You need to become accustomed to eating a balanced breakfast with protein, fat, and carbohydrates. Eating breakfast revs up your metabolism for the day. After a while, you will become hungry for breakfast, and your metabolism will benefit.

Boosting Your Metabolism

You've probably heard that it's important to keep your metabolism high to lose weight. You don't have to settle for living with a slow metabolism. Wishing and hoping won't enhance your metabolic rate, but doing the right things will. Here are effective ways to boost your metabolism and keep it high throughout your life:

♦ Make sure that you do not inadvertently put yourself into starvation metabolism. If you do, correct the situation as soon as you can.

♦ Avoid overeating because this stalls the efficient burning of fuel. Eat from 0–5. Overeating forces the body to store more fat, increasing your body fat percentage. This slows your metabolism.

♦ Increase the muscle percentage in your body and decrease your body fat percentage. The higher the muscle mass, the faster you burn fuel. As you increase muscle mass, your basal metabolic rate increases. Do this with two to three sessions of strength-training exercise a week. Use free weights, weight machines, Pilates, or exercises with flex bands or the Fitness Ball. You'll love how your body looks with more muscle and less body fat.

Body of Knowledge

An equivalent weight of muscle is one third the size of fat. As you increase muscle mass percentage, you will be smaller and fit into those jeans.

◆ Don't severely limit your intake of proteins, fats, or carbohydrates. Eat balanced meals so that your body has enough nutrition to keep your metabolism high.

◆ Get plenty of sleep every night. Not getting enough sleep slows your metabolism.

◆ Use the power of your mind to propel yourself to a higher metabolic rate. Tell yourself that you have a high metabolism. Also be sure to keep saying aloud to yourself that you are at your ideal size. You'll learn more about this in Part 6.

◆ Avoid continually running on adrenaline or living with a chronic stress situation. Reduce or eliminate stress with the stress-soothing suggestions in Chapter 8.

◆ Breathe deeply. Get plenty of oxygen. For fuel to burn, it needs lots of oxygen. Get this from exercise and from taking deep breaths that you can feel all the way into your stomach. This is called diaphragm breathing.

◆ Don't skip meals. When you're hungry, eat 0–5.

◆ Consider alcohol to be a food and factor it into your overall food consumption.

◆ Avoid watching TV or playing video or computer games for more than a couple hours at a time. When you watch television, your body's metabolism drops almost to sleeping levels. When we sleep, our metabolic rate is the lowest of the day.

◆ Just as you should only eat when you are hungry, only sip on sweet-tasting liquids when you are hungry, or at 0 on the hunger scale. This includes juices and beverages sweetened with artificial sweeteners, such as diet sodas, as well as beverages sweetened with sugar or honey.

◆ Drink plenty of water—at least eight glasses a day. Being hydrated increases your metabolism.

These guidelines are used throughout this book as we discuss foods, exercise, and diet programs. We strongly encourage you to use these criteria to help you lose weight and keep it off. If your weight-loss plan violates these guidelines, you won't get the results you desire.

The Least You Need to Know

- If your eating habits swing between deprivation and excess, your body goes into starvation metabolism and stores fat.

- Your metabolism and basal metabolic rate are influenced by your lifestyle decisions.

- In starvation metabolism, your body instinctively hoards fat out of fear that it will eventually face deprivation or famine, and this slows your metabolism way down.

- You can avoid starvation metabolism by eating when you are hungry. On the hunger scale, eat when your stomach is at 0 and stop when you are at 5 or below.

- Balanced-eating food plans let you avoid starvation metabolism.

- Limit your intake of caffeine to meals and snack-times.

Chapter 7

Eating Beautifully and Sensuously

In This Chapter

♦ Learn eating behaviors that make you thin

♦ Mealtime is for relaxation and enjoyment

♦ Here's to your good digestion

Having a weight issue typically means having a love-hate affair with food. You might love to eat but hate what food does to your body and self-esteem. This love-hate affair makes mealtimes challenging. You just can't seem to approach food in a simple, satisfying way. You're not alone.

In this chapter, we'll reveal how to turn your relationship with food into a love-love affair. We'll explore how to get the most out of every delicious bite, while at the same time eating so that your body benefits the most from your food. Food will become your friend … *not* your enemy and *not* an object of unbridled desire!

The Pleasure of Food

Eating is truly one of life's most pleasurable and sensuous activities. Quite simply, food tastes good. It pleases all your senses of taste. Food offers delightful aromas and textures. It refreshes us. Enjoying food, especially delicious food, is one of the most natural experiences in the world. Hooray!

So why do we persist in our love-hate relationship with food? It's so unnecessary. Food in and of itself cannot make you fat. It has no such power. The power resides in you and your eating habits. If you overeat any food, you can gain weight. If you eat food using the 0–5 approach described in Chapter 5, you can reach your ideal size.

A Healthy Appetite Really Is Healthy

Just as hunger is a valuable feeling you don't want to suppress, a normal appetite is a good thing, too. Appetite is the desire for food. Your normal appetite for certain foods fluctuates from day to day. You should honor your appetite. Don't ignore or resist its natural function. For instance, you might have an appetite for eggs and bacon for breakfast. You don't have to resist your appetite and eat only cereal. Go ahead and eat the eggs and bacon.

Crazy About Those Cravings

Unfortunately, there is such a thing as a false appetite. A false appetite is basically an irrational craving. Your brain becomes self-programmed to desire something so strongly that it incites you to compulsive consumption. Your false appetite often is for foods that can be harmful, such as allergic foods, lots of sugar, and highly processed refined starches such as breads, pasta, cookies, and cakes. We call these *fluffy starches*.

Mike, a college student, is allergic to wheat, corn, and milk products. They give him stomach cramps and frequent diarrhea. He can't resist eating certain wheat products, especially sandwich bread … even when it makes him sick. His craving for bread can be so extreme that he will even put a fancy steak between two pieces of bread with a couple slices of cheese. Like someone who needs a daily fix of coffee, his desire for bread compels him to eat irrationally. His eating habits are ruining his fun and health. Of course, he can ultimately control his urge for these allergic foods by substituting other foods he loves that aren't harmful.

You can manage your appetite by directing it toward good-for-you foods such as the basics—meat, fruits, vegetables, and fats. If one day you have an urge for broccoli, give in to it. Ditto for steak, salmon, salad, and so on. Your body will be glad you did. You don't need to battle your appetite. Just manage it as one part of your overall eating approach.

Good Digestion Comes with Pleasurable Eating

Many people who are overweight have poor digestion. For the most part, poor digestion is not inherited or genetic. We give it to ourselves through the way we eat. Eating to soothe stress or anxiety is often the culprit.

Alas, poor digestion can lead to weight problems. Here's how: When a person feels stressed, the part of the central nervous system that regulates digestion switches off. This is called the parasympathetic nervous system. At those times of stress, the body can take in food and process some of it, but digestion doesn't work correctly to extract all the nutritional goodness from the food.

Poor digestion is not always obvious by observing symptoms. You could get heartburn, diarrhea, or constipation, but not always. Poor digestion can be seemingly silent.

If you eat when you are stressed, anxious, or nervous, you might as well be eating cardboard for all the nutrients your body gets. Yes, eating when stressed is a gaining situation. Now you might think, well, gosh, if I'm not digesting, the calories aren't getting handled, so I should be losing weight. Good idea, but wrong reality. When digestion is impaired, the body starts "starving" from lack of necessary nutrients. Yes, it goes into starvation metabolism and starts hoarding fat and energy. It thinks it's in a famine. The good news is that it's easy to make some corrections and get rid of stress at mealtimes.

If you feel stressed often, it can be helpful to take a supplement that contains multiple B vitamins. These help, but you could still find yourself stressed at mealtimes. Here's how to make meals a pleasant "losing" experience.

Eating with Elegance and Grace

Whether you're eating hamburgers on the patio, a hot dog at a baseball game, or a five-course dinner on Valentine's Day, you can use the following principles of eating with elegance and grace. Yes, even if you are eating with babies and small children, you can improve your digestion and enjoy your meal.

Eat Beautifully

Think back to your eating environments for the past three or four days. Have you eaten in the car, in front of the TV, or with your e-mail as a companion? Have you eaten at your desk or during a difficult and emotional discussion? Have you been so upset that you took your dinner to bed with you? In each situation, you're missing an opportunity to eat beautifully and healthfully. Eating beautifully means eating in an environment that is peaceful, health-giving, and enjoyable.

Let's start with the basics. Beautiful eating is eating while seated at a table with utensils, plates, and napkins, maybe even with placemats or a tablecloth. Even better, include flowers, candles, and perhaps a centerpiece.

Next think about the sounds you want to hear when you are enjoying your food. Do you want to hear the evening news, a TV sitcom, or an argument the children are waging? Or do you want lovely music and even better conversation? You will enjoy eating—and will eat more intelligently—if you turn off the TV and focus on your food and your eating companions. Stop reading and just enjoy your food. If the phone rings, you don't need to answer it. That's what voice messaging is for—to handle phone calls when you don't want to. The phone ringing is not a good enough reason to interrupt your enjoyment of your food. Food is such a wonderful thing in and of itself that you don't need a diversion. In fact, it's so wonderful that it deserves your full attention.

In a study of women, some ate while watching an interesting suspense story on television. The others simply ate their food without outside stimulation. The second group ate less food at the meal than those who watched the show.

The most fattening eating can be done when standing up or lying down. How many of us have shoveled in lots of food while standing in front of the kitchen sink staring out the window? Far too many. Eating while sitting sounds so fundamental. People who are at their ideal size are not the people who hover over the hors d'oeuvres at a cocktail buffet. They don't eat a full dinner while standing at the stove cooking dinner. Most adults who are at their ideal size enjoy beautiful meals. So whenever you are hungry, sit down and eat. Don't stand and stuff.

> **CAUTION**
>
> ### Weighty Warning
>
> One of our clients got distressed whenever she didn't receive a scheduled phone call from her boyfriend. Her solution was to order a pizza and take it to bed. Eating to soothe emotions while lying in bed is fattening and not beautiful or sensuous.

The best way to practice this principle of sitting to eat is to take all of your food and snacks to your place at the dining room or kitchen table. Eat your food there.

Eat Calmly

What have you brought with you to the meal? Set aside your concerns of the day when you sit down to eat. Believe us, they will be right where you left them when the meal is over. You can set guidelines for conversations at dinner. If someone insists on discussing things you don't want to hear about, you can put your fork down and wait until the person stops. You never need to eat even one mouthful of food in an environment or situation you don't like. Should your children act up, as children often do, put your fork down until the ruckus abates. There's no reason to ruin good food by eating it in chaos.

You have the opportunity for three or more pleasurable eating interludes every day. Don't let them get messed up with less-than-pleasurable surroundings and activities. As best you can, eat beautifully at every meal. Yes, we know you can't always do this. But whenever you can and as often as you can, make your meals beautiful.

Slow Down and Lose Weight

By eating slowly, you give your stomach the best chance for good digestion. For several reasons, a meal should take at least 15 minutes. Twenty minutes or longer is better yet.

It takes about 15 minutes from the time when you begin eating for your stomach to signal the brain that it has had enough food and that it is satisfied and comfortable. Your mouth can consume food faster than your stomach can register that you have eaten it.

If you eat quickly, you are more likely to overeat, easily reaching 6 or higher on the 0–10 scale. It is difficult to eat beautifully and sensuously in less than 15 minutes.

> **Thinspiration**
>
> Do you savor every mouthful of food you eat? Enjoying the taste of every bite is very helpful in limiting the quantity of food you consume. Eat slowly and be sure to chew each bite and swallow before you take the next bite.

Chew Sanely

We are often asked how many times a person should chew before swallowing. Rather than answer this question directly—we don't want you to ruin your meal by counting chews—we prefer to think of it this way. Finish swallowing what is already in your mouth before you take the next bite. Before you swallow, chew thoroughly and slowly. Eating is not a race you win if you eat the fastest. Make every mouthful a delight.

Chewing is the first step in the digestive process. Saliva starts to break down the food and prepare it for the stomach. If you bypass chewing, your digestive efficiency is impaired.

The Least You Need to Know

- Make your eating a pleasurable experience; you will eat less food and be more satisfied.

- Eat slowly and eat seated, making sure to take at least 15 minutes per meal or snack.

- At mealtime, turn off the television and simply enjoy your food.

Chapter **8**

Stress, Eating, and You

In This Chapter

- How stress can make you fat
- Mastering stress before it controls you
- The perils of eating when stressed
- Great ways to soothe stress

Losing unwanted weight will probably make you happier. Guess what? Staying happier will also help you lose weight! That's because ordinary day-to-day stress can inhibit your weight-loss program's effectiveness. That's probably no surprise to you. Stress affects us both physically and psychologically. Stress eating adds pounds, and stress all by itself even without overeating can add inches to your waistline.

Do the following situations sound familiar? It's a Friday night and you're feeling blue, so you munch your way through a bag of Oreos. Or you come home from work wound up like a ball of string and gobble a hefty piece of cake … before dinner! Or you sit down to lunch or dinner while taking care of paperwork and practically slurp down your meal without tasting it. You are stress eating. It's time to break the stress eating bad habits.

Running on Adrenaline Is Fattening

Living in a state of chronic and relentless stress actually adds pounds, regardless of what you are eating. You can have a very sound food plan and exercise regimen, and your best intentions can get derailed because of stress.

Frank is a businessman who worked in a major city, but a few years ago he moved his family to a pastoral location 40 miles away. His morning and afternoon commutes were at least an hour long, even longer if there was snow or ice on the roads. By nature, Frank was a pretty high-intensity person, and the commutes made him even more tense and anxious. After a year, Frank's weight had increased 40 pounds, most of it around his middle. The commutes were ruining his dream of enjoying the countryside, so Frank and his family moved back to the city. His commute time dropped to about 15 to 20 minutes. Within six months, he lost the extra weight without altering his eating in any way.

During the long, congested, and sometimes treacherous commute, Frank's body instinctively shifted into fight-or-flight mode. Subconsciously, he was on ready alert and his *adrenaline* was working overtime. Even Stone Age men didn't have to run away from the woolly mammoth every single morning and evening five days a week for one to two hours! Yikes! While Frank's automobile ran on gas, he ran on adrenaline. He was under chronic stress.

When stress causes adrenaline to be secreted into the blood stream, along with it comes cortisol, a hormone that is responsible for putting on waistline weight. Recent research shows that when our bodies produce too much cortisol, we gain weight with or without eating changes.

Lean Lingo

Adrenaline is a hormone that directly affects the brain as a stimulus and indirectly affects our entire body. Our primitive ancestors relied on adrenaline for survival. An adrenal hormone, cortisol, causes weight gain around the waist and midsection. To get rid of the "spare tire" waist, reduce the chronic stress in your life and get enough sleep.

Frank didn't move back to the city to lose weight; he just wanted more quality time with his family. He wanted more time ... period. But a wonderful side benefit was that his weight returned to normal. By simply changing his home address, he consequently changed his weight.

If you can find a way to change your lifestyle to reduce stress significantly, do it. You will find that your weight issues will improve or dissolve. Unfortunately, sometimes making the change doesn't seem feasible, as was the case with Laura.

Laura was an executive with a Fortune 100 company. Because of her work, most weeks she traveled from Sunday evening through Friday evening. Appointments were preset for her every day. She typically started her day with a breakfast meeting with one customer, called on customers all day long, and then ended the day with a customer dinner meeting. Her Friday dinner was often a not-exactly-gourmet meal on yet one more airplane flying home. On weekends, she did laundry, slept, and prepared for the next week.

Laura never enjoyed down time. She ran on adrenaline, not just three hours a day but virtually full time, day after day. She got by on just enough sleep, zonking out after finishing her business dinner and catching up on e-mails. She slept hard until the hotel wakeup call signaled that it was time to get ready for another customer breakfast. Laura was about 65 pounds overweight, and most of it was around her tummy. No weight-loss program had ever worked for her since she'd accepted her well-paying executive position.

Was it possible for Laura to slow the adrenaline rush? Absolutely. But it didn't seem possible to her. She could have used relaxation techniques such as exercising at the hotel's exercise facility before breakfast and enjoying a warm bath every night before bed. By also being attentive to eating 0–5, Laura could have released her adrenaline-cortisol weight.

> **Weighty Warning**
>
> When a person drinks beer and other alcoholic beverages, the body releases the hormone cortisol, which causes weight gain around the waist. They aren't called beer bellies for nothing!

Running on Adrenaline Is Like Running on a Treadmill

So what good is cortisol? It's the key actor in the second part of a three-phase stress cycle. Phase one is the release of adrenaline, the fight-or-flight hormone. This happens when we are faced with imminent danger. Adrenaline gives us a quick energy jolt. Phase 2 is the release of cortisol, sometimes called the master strategist. Cortisol helps us think fast and creatively and make good life-saving decisions. Phase 3 is the recovery phase, a time in which the stress hormones leave our bodies and we get back to normal.

The problem today is that many people never move on to phase 3. Instead, they move from one stressful situation to the next, and their cortisol levels remain high continuously.

Cortisol served our primitive ancestors in another fundamental way. It helped them store fat. When we run on adrenaline, cortisol helps our bodies create new fat cells so that we'll have enough stored energy to give us a boost when needed. The bodies of both Frank and Laura got signals—completely unconsciously—from the cortisol rushing through their blood to store fat … just in case the fat would be needed for a later energy boost.

Are you running on adrenaline and cortisol too much? Work isn't the only culprit. Raising small children is often a fattening time in many women's lives. Although many women thrive in the milieu of motherhood, others get stressed out from the continual demands of small children and household management. Despite the need to rush around, take care of everyone, and only snatch a bite to eat here and there, moms often still put on pounds! It might not seem fair, but remember, a little self-TLC—like a hot bath—will be good for you … and everyone else in the family.

You know whether the stress in your life is too much. Look carefully at your life and figure out how to cut back on stress. You will likely be cutting back on your weight problem, too.

"Stressed" Spelled Backward Is "Desserts"

In times of anxiety, sadness, boredom, or nervousness, an overeater traipses off to the kitchen. The foods in the pantry or refrigerator seem to offer instant relief. She indulges her need for the pastries, cakes, cookies, crackers, and other yummy starches that will take away the bad feelings.

For someone with a weight issue, stress and eating usually go together like cream cheese on a bagel. They seem meant for each other. You wouldn't believe how many "confessions" we've heard about eating an entire bag of cookies or a carton of ice cream to soothe stress!

Those who don't seek out food when stressed cannot understand this habit. They listen to music, take a walk, or call a friend when they're out of sorts. But eat snack foods? "Why would I do that?" they ask. If you're a stress eater, however, you're probably right now shaking your head in disbelief that not everyone tries to eat away their blues.

Ever wonder why you don't gobble up steak and green beans at stressful moments? Because they don't work. They are just plain ordinary food. For most of us, steak and green beans don't have that magic something that elevates mood and temporarily anesthetizes the eater.

Starches like cookies, cakes, and crackers are definitely mood elevators, and they counter-act the depressing effect cortisol has on brain neurotransmitters. They increase *serotonin* levels in the brain, chemically altering a person's mood and giving the eater a lift. In a sense, eating starches is not a bad choice when you are having a bad moment. Starches work. They make you feel better and are cheap. What's not to like? The answer: what they do to your body and self-esteem. They will make you gain weight when you overeat them.

> **Lean Lingo**
>
> **Serotonin** is a natural neurotransmitter in the brain that lifts mood. When we eat highly starchy foods such as cakes, cookies, bagels, and chips, more serotonin is released into the brain, and we feel soothed. **Stress soothers** are positive, inspiring, and uplifting alternatives to use when you're tempted to eat to soothe stress.

Beating the Blues without Feeding Your Face

Breaking the bad mood–munchies cycle is relatively easy after you find a great alternative to relieve stress. In surveying hundreds of overweight people about what works for them to soothe their anxieties and depression blues, we've come up with a list of excellent alternatives. The criteria for acceptance into our Stress Soothers Hall of Fame were demanding.

Stress soothers had to be all of the following: legal, inexpensive, accessible (able to do at the office or simply by ducking into the nearest bathroom), nonfattening, positive, inspiring, uplifting, practical, realistic, quick, and solitary (can be done by yourself).

The suggestions that didn't make the Stress Soothers Hall of Fame were meditation and jogging. Meditation is a great idea, but it's not practical for most people at the moment of frantically needing to soothe stress. But if you meditate regularly, go for it. And jogging works great if you don't have small children at home, but typically is not what a stress eater would do or would want to do. But if you do love to jog, put your shoes on and go banish your stress.

The key to a good stress soother is that it redirects your interests away from the kitchen while it provides you with relaxation and a reduction in cortisol stress levels.

Simple and Effective Stress Soothers

Researchers can measure a person's cortisol levels through a simple saliva test. In research settings, they ask a group of people to relax on a sofa while watching television for an hour. The researchers measured before and after cortisol rates. The verdict: watching television didn't lower cortisol levels. Later in their research they conducted a similar experiment but substituted an hour of yoga for watching television. You guessed it. The group's cortisol levels were significantly reduced.

In the following list, you won't find watching television as a stress soother. What you will find are activities that lower your cortisol levels. You're certain to find one or two that work for you during stressful times. They'll lift your moods and make you forget you ever considered a cookie fling just to make yourself feel better.

Get in Water

Water works. Take a bath, take a shower, get in the hot tub, or go swimming. Warm water envelops the largest organ of the body, the skin. It warms up every pore and relaxes the muscles.

When I (Lucy) was losing my weight more than 20 years ago, I took baths long before I intellectually understood them. The most difficult overeating time of day for me was late afternoon. I found water to be the perfect relaxant. When I could get my hyperactive 3-year-old son to take a nap, I would hustle to the bathroom and enjoy a bubble bath. These were not necessarily long, luxurious baths; my son was likely to need me at any moment. Sometimes I took three-minute baths; sometimes they lasted for five minutes. But they worked.

I imagined that all the stress in me was going into the water and down the drain. By the time I put on fresh clothes, the urge to eat had subsided, and I looked forward to the rest of the day. Today, my grown-up son comments on how many baths I took when he was a baby. You bet, I say; they made me thin.

Get Warm

We are not bears. We don't need to add on a layer of fat to carry us through the winter, but some of us are inclined to add winter weight. When physically chilled or cold, we're prone to eat more starches. You don't need to add pounds in winter to get more warmth. Wear clothes that are warmer and, when you feel chilled, put on your flannel PJs, get under the down comforter, and sip on a cup of warm herbal or decaffeinated tea. Getting warm can also soothe bad feelings.

Get in the Sunshine

Sunshine is the perfect mood lifter. Research indicates that 20 minutes of sunlight a day will naturally elevate your mood. Twenty minutes of sunshine daily also helps your hormones work correctly. People who live in the northernmost states or in areas of the country with lots of rainy days are often deficient in sunlight. The ensuing depression is called seasonal affective disorder (SAD). It can be remedied by exposure to plenty of natural sunlight or by using artificial full-spectrum bright light, as provided by a *light box*. Sources for purchasing light boxes can be found in Appendix B.

It's best to get real sunshine. You can do this even if you work indoors. Eat lunch on the patio, take a walk during break time, or play outdoors with the children when you get home from work.

For your 20 minutes of sun therapy a day, wear sunscreen but don't wear your sunglasses. Your eyes need the light to boost hormonal activity and elevate your moods. Of course, never look directly at the sun; instead, simply sit, walk, garden, or relax.

Lean Lingo

A **light box** is a clever device that mimics natural full-spectrum sunlight. A small one stands about 16 inches wide and less than 2 feet high. It can sit on a desk or hang on a wall. Sitting in front of the box for even a half-hour a day can perk you up on wintry or cloudy days.

Dry Brush Your Body

Purchase a natural-bristle brush or loofah from the drugstore or a discount store. Some are designed for dry-brushing the skin. The brush shouldn't be too stiff or too soft. With long strokes, dry brush your body. Start at your feet and work up your legs to your torso. Brush your tummy and buttocks. Then brush your arms, starting with your hands and working up to your shoulders. If you have a long-handled brush, brush your back. Finish up with brushing your chest and neck.

You will love this. It is so invigorating. It seems to make your body feel alive and refreshed. It can lift your mood. Dry brush your body before you shower in the morning or at any time of day when you feel a need to de-stress.

Although we recommend dry brushing your body for its mood-elevating effects, it also has some terrific health benefits. When you dry brush the body, you're assisting the lymph system in removing toxins. After a couple of weeks, you might notice that your skin is smoother and that even slight imperfections are gone. People who have done this for years report having skin like a baby.

Brush Your Hair

Doesn't brushing your hair sound almost too simple? Don't let its simplicity fool you. Clients rave about its effectiveness. The best hairbrush for this technique is very inexpensive. Purchase the kind that has rough plastic bristles. The brushes with the fancy rounded tips don't work well. We purchase ours at the discount chains.

To brush your hair, bend over from the waist and brush so that you can feel the bristles on your scalp. Brush enthusiastically for a minute or so and then stand up. Your scalp will tingle and will feel as though you are massaging your brain chemicals directly. We doubt this actually happens, but it sure feels that way. It's also great for your hair and scalp.

Just imagine, in just a couple of minutes of brushing, you could brush away the stress-induced urge to eat.

The Back Roller Rolls Away Your Stress

The back roller is wooden and looks like a rolling pin with waves in it. The waves correspond to your spine and to the erector muscles on either side of your spine.

Use the back roller to roll away your stress.

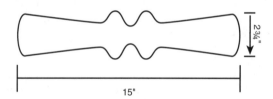

Lie face up with your spine in the middle dip of the roller. Beginning just below the neck, slowly move the roller from one vertebra to the next going down the spine. At each vertebra, breathe about 10 breaths and let your erector muscles on either side of the spine relax. It takes about 10 to 15 minutes to move all the way down the spine. By this time, you'll be blissfully and totally relaxed. The urge to eat will have evaporated. When you stand up, your posture will be better, you'll look taller, and you'll be relaxed. Count on it.

Carry the back roller with you when you travel. It soothes the aches and pains caused by sitting on airplanes. Some aficionados claim it keeps their backs in alignment. Others applaud how it stimulates acupressure points for all the major organs and glands of the body on its path down the spine. Others rave that it drains the lymph nodes on either side of the spine. Some claim it soothes their aching backs.

You can purchase a back roller at health-food stores and specialty stores that carry products for back care. It's inexpensive and lasts a lifetime. Information about purchasing a back roller online is in Appendix B.

Having a Ball on a Ball

Body rolling is incomparable for deep muscle relaxation. You can body roll at home and perhaps even in the office if you can shut your door during a break. By simply resting your body weight on different-sized balls, depending on which part of the body you're relaxing, the muscles close to the bone as well as the larger muscles relax. You can roll down the thighs and calves. You can roll up the spine and then roll up each side of the spine for a total of three times rolling up the back. You can include rolling up your abdomen. Use a smaller ball about the size of a tennis ball to roll on the soles of your feet.

It is best to have plenty of quiet time for body rolling so that you can experience deep relaxation over every nook and cranny of your body. The good news is that you can enjoy body rolling while watching the children or talking on the phone if need be.

Body rolling your entire body in one session would be too intense. Instead, choose a different part for each session. We love body rolling first for relaxation. However, we have noticed improved posture and less cellulite. Where and how to purchase the balls with instructions can be found in Appendix B.

Sing Away Your Stress

As I was sharing the Stress Soothers Hall of Fame selections with my husband, he said, "Lucy, you forgot to tell them about the Stones." I hadn't a clue what he was talking about. He said, "You know, the Stones. Every time the Rolling Stones come on the radio, your brain chemistry changes. You start dancing and singing along."

Your favorite music might not be the Rolling Stones, but there's probably certain music that makes you feel great. Maybe it's a favorite rock group from your youth or perhaps classical music. Maybe it's the Beatles, Beethoven, disco, or U2. Keep your favorite tunes handy, and when the bad feelings come that make you want to dive into starches, turn on your music and sing along. So don't sing for your supper; instead, sing for your ideal size.

Hobbies and Games

Do you have a hobby, craft, or puzzle that you can pick up when you need to relax? Activities such as knitting, needlepoint, or crossword puzzles can so totally engage your hands and your mind that you cannot eat at the same time. A difficult solitaire game or a computer game may be all you need to get your energy headed in a new direction.

A half-hour or even 15 minutes of knitting can soothe and refresh you. Ditto a craft that you love. Whatever it is, however, you need to keep it accessible at a moment's notice. Unfortunately, gardening is one hobby that you can't do as easily year round, but it's great during the planting and growing seasons.

Other possible activities in this category include reading magazines, polishing silver, art projects, journaling, and playing a musical instrument. If you have a piano that's mostly gathering dust, tap on those ivories as a way to divert the blues.

Cortisol-Lowering Supplements

Yes, you can take dietary supplements that naturally block or lower cortisol levels. They work especially well to soothe you, and as an added benefit, they can help whittle fat stored in your mid-section. You'll still need to eat 0–5 and eat well nutritionally.

- ◆ Theanine. Our personal favorite. Theanine is an inexpensive supplement available at the health-food store. This non-essential amino acid is found in green and black tea. It works within 20 minutes to soothe you for about 2 hours, while it increases alpha brain waves—the ones that make you mentally sharp, relaxed, and awake. It's quite safe. You can take it three times a day or only when you need some calming.

- ◆ Mixed herbals. You'll find combinations of ingredients such as magnolia bark, epimedium, phytoterols, phosphatidylserine, tyrosine, and others. If you find one that gives you good results, use it when you need some help relaxing. As of now, all of these ingredients are thought to be safe.

- ◆ Supplements specially designed for weight loss. Use caution when trying any of these. Sometimes the formulations include ingredients that hype up your metabolism while the other ingredients soothe you.

Supplements aren't the entire answer to reducing stress, but are helpful. Use a variety of stress soothers to master stress.

Long-Term Solutions to Short-Term Stress

The following activities might not work instantly, but over time they will help you reduce stress and the urge to consume serotonin-releasing starches.

Regular Massages. If you can afford massages, go for it. Even one massage every two to three weeks soothes ongoing daily stress. Massages ease tight muscles and can help the body detoxify through hand manipulation of the muscles and lymph nodes.

Stretch Away the Stress and Cravings. A regular program of stretching reduces stress. Stretching releases built-up body tension. Stretch regularly, about three times a week. That way, you can release the stress held in muscles before it adds fat to those muscles.

Stretching is a great option at home and in many semiprivate places. Many health clubs offer *yoga*, *Pilates*, and stretching classes. Excellent books and videos are available on stretching techniques. You'll learn more in Part 4.

Lean Lingo

Yoga and **Pilates** are excellent forms of exercise for strengthening, stretching, and balance. Both techniques help you de-stress because they engage the mind as well as the body. Yoga originated in India many thousands of years ago, and Pilates was created by Joseph Pilates about 50 years ago. Pilates exercises create flexibility and overall strength to build long, lean, strong, and fluid bodies. The exercises might seem familiar, such as a sit-up or leg lift, but the execution is slower and more focused on posture and abdominal control than other exercise systems. More information about each approach is available in Part 4.

Aerobicize Away Your Stress. One significant benefit of aerobic exercise is often overlooked—*endorphin* release. Endorphins are chemical agents released into the blood stream that make your brain feel good. Endorphins are released from several kinds of activities, including vigorous exercise, sex, and laughter. They're also released when we eat fatty foods, like chocolate and cheesecake, and starches, such as breads, cookies, and potatoes.

By doing enough aerobic exercise, even as little as 20 minutes daily, your body releases endorphins that make you feel good all over and that override the feelings of bad moods and anxiety.

Meditation, Contemplation, and Prayer. Meditation, contemplation, and prayer are spiritual activities that can help sooth your stress. When practiced often, preferably daily, they keep you focused on the big picture of your life. If any one of these suit you, practice it on a consistent basis. You'll reap countless rewards.

Here are a couple "extras" that can reduce your stress level without adding weight:

- **Herbal teas.** Make sure these don't contain caffeine. Hot chamomile tea relaxes lots of folks, but you might prefer another flavor.

- **Water.** Preferably purified, hot or cold. Drink it slowly.

- **Aromatherapy.** Fill your room with the delightful scents of essential oils that soothe, such as lavender, jasmine, or clary sage.

You can use all of these remedies for stress when low moods send you to the refrigerator or cookie jar. Try them on for size and determine the ones that work best for you. Do one of the stress soothers before you head for the mood-altering starches. Stress soothers are great for you in many ways—for your health, your mental attitude, your relaxation, and best of all, attaining your ideal size.

The Least You Need to Know

- Chronic stress causes weight gain around the waist.

- Eliminate chronic stress by changing your circumstances if possible.

- Use stress-soothing techniques daily to reduce cortisol levels and stress.

- Cortisol-lowering supplements can help you with stress management.

- To reduce stress in your life, take a proactive approach through daily activities that ease stress buildup.

Part  3

Food Supports Your Weight Loss

This part of the book is about food. After all, you've got to eat, and you won't get to your ideal size by not eating. In fact, eating well is essential to reaching your ideal size and staying there for life. In this part, you'll read straightforward explanations of the essential qualities of proteins, carbs, fats, and other nutrients such as vitamins and minerals and how to balance them in a safe, nutritious eating plan. When you're finished, you'll come away with simple, practical guidelines that help you choose foods and prepare meals wisely ... while attaining and maintaining your ideal size.

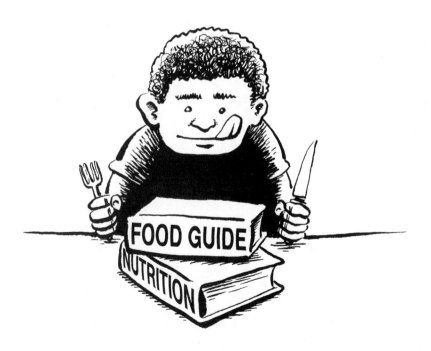

Proteins, Fats, and Carbohydrates

In This Chapter

- The importance of protein for weight loss
- Fats are essential for weight loss
- Your good health depends on eating the right fat
- Eating carbohydrates to reduce fat stores

For all of the many different foods you've eaten and enjoyed, they all fall into one of three categories. Actually four, if you count artificial substances, such as diet sodas, and artificial sweeteners, which we don't count as food.

And the three categories are proteins (such as meats, fish, poultry, eggs, and cheese), fats (such as butter and olive oil), and carbohydrates (such as fruits and vegetables). The realm of carbohydrates is quite large because it also contains grains, sugars, and the fluffy white treats we know and love all too well—the cakes, cookies, donuts, white potatoes, and breads.

In this chapter, you'll learn the importance of each for optimal nutrition and weight loss.

Protein Means Power and a Whole Lot More

In our world of fast foods and convenience foods, eating high-quality protein can be hard to do. Yet without protein, your hair could fall out, your fingernails could crumble, and your muscles could deteriorate into, well, mush. You are unlikely to reach your ideal size—and stay energetic—without a steady diet of high-quality protein.

Think about it. In the right quantities, steak is really good for you! So are almost all lean meats, eggs, and cheeses. Proteins give you energy, and your body needs them to manufacture hormones, antibodies, enzymes, and tissues. Your body cannot be healthy without the essential *amino acids* found in protein. They're called "essential" because your body can't manufacture them on its own. You need a regular dose of essential amino acids in your diet. Yes, your body needs "nonessential" amino acids, but it can synthesize them.

Lean Lingo

Amino acids are called the "building blocks of life." Protein from food is digested into amino acids. The amino acids are used to build and maintain muscles and other tissues. They are also important in enzyme and hormone production.

After water, protein makes up the largest portion of your body weight. This includes muscles, ligaments, tendons, organs, glands, nails, and hair. Protein is needed in your diet so that your body is healthy and functions properly.

Essential and Nonessential Amino Acids

The essential amino acids can be obtained only by consuming certain protein-containing foods. They are histidine, isoleucine, leucine, lysine, methionine, phenylalanine, threonine, tryptophan, and valine. All of the other amino acids are nonessential, meaning that they are manufactured in the body. In fact, some are created from the aforementioned essential amino acids.

In the simplest of terms, all of this translates to one critical point: you need to eat protein. So how do you select which proteins to add to your eating plan?

Complete or Incomplete, Take Your Pick

Protein-containing foods come in two versions:

- *Complete proteins* contain all the essential amino acids. These proteins are found in meats, fish, seafood, poultry, eggs, and dairy.

♦ *Incomplete proteins* contain only some of the essential amino acids. Foods with incomplete protein include grains, legumes, nuts, seeds, and some leafy vegetables. Soybean products, such as tofu, tempeh, and soy protein isolate are not complete proteins because they're low or deficient in methionine.

Some individuals have difficulty digesting protein because their bodies don't secrete sufficient proteases and hydrochloric acid. Clues that you might not be digesting protein well include soft, peeling, or splitting fingernails or a heavy, unpleasant feeling after eating protein. Certain dietary supplements, discussed in Chapter 11, can help.

Lean Lingo

Complete proteins are foods that contain balanced amounts of all the essential amino acids that the human body needs to build and repair muscle and body organs. These are the animal proteins, such as meat, fish, eggs, and cheese. **Incomplete proteins** contain only some of the essential amino acids, but could offer nutritional value. These include soy, legumes, and grain. **Food combining** means eating more than one incomplete protein at a meal, which could provide adequate protein, but may not.

Combining Incomplete Proteins into Complete Proteins

Food combining is a way to eat incomplete proteins so that you get all the essential amino acids. You can combine legumes such as pinto beans, black beans, navy beans, and lentils with grains, such as rice, corn, and wheat or with nuts and seeds.

Food combining isn't your best source of complete protein. You'll be able to lose weight more easily when you eat animal protein at each meal. But on occasion, you can use food combining for variety.

Weight-Loss Benefits of Protein

By eating complete protein at every meal, you give yourself nutritional support to keep your energy high until your next meal. Proteins provide critical components your body needs for fat burning. The most common tendency of people who don't eat enough protein for breakfast is to crash during mid- to late afternoon. They then overeat the quick, pick-me-up, high-glycemic starches and sugars. This is a sure way to gain rather than lose weight.

Your Basic Protein Requirements

An average-sized woman needs about 15 to 21 grams of complete protein at each meal. An average-sized man needs about 20 to 28 grams, based on eating three meals a day. That's about 3 ounces of meat or fish for a woman and 4 ounces for a man. Three ounces of meat is about the size of a small mini can of tuna or the size of a deck of cards. If you eat a protein snack, lower the grams of protein you eat at regular meals.

Low Blood Sugar Be Gone

When you eat the recommended amount of protein at each meal, chronic low blood sugar can be a thing of your past. Far too many people get stuck in yo-yo eating, starving themselves one moment and then eating high-glycemic-loaded meals when their energy is gone.

You are less likely to have your hunger numbers drop below 0 when you eat at least 15 grams or 3 ounces of complete protein for breakfast, lunch, and dinner. That's not to say that eating protein completely solves low blood sugar. Proper eating of fats and carbohydrates also helps.

Some low-blood-sugar situations for women are also associated with hormonal cycles. You might experience the effects of low blood sugar in the days prior to your menstrual period even when you eat balanced meals including protein, but they should become lulls and not crashes.

Fats Can Make You Thin

Eating fat is essential to reaching your ideal size. Fats do not, as a friend recently suggested at lunch, go directly from one's mouth to the fat cells on the tummy and hips. Of course, anyone who overeats fat could gain weight. Some is great for weight loss—too much isn't. Over and over again, when our fat-phobic clients add fat back into their eating, their stubborn weight starts coming off. So get ready to eat *some* fat and reach your ideal size!

Fats Are Not the Enemy

Dietary fat is an important component of a healthy diet. By eating the right fats in the right proportions, you can enjoy watching your body fat melt away.

Before we get into some of the nitty-gritty details about dietary fat, let's list some of the known benefits of fat:

- Fat is required to manufacture hormones. Without fat, your hormones get out of whack. This includes your thyroid and the regulation of women's hormonal cycles, including menopause and conception. Men require optimum hormonal activity for high-energy sex and good muscle mass.

- Fats are required for the proper communication of the neurotransmitters in the brain.

- Fat is necessary for many metabolic processes such as red blood cell formation and *insulin* functions.

- Fat lubricates your joints, maintains healthy skin, and aids in the digestion process.

Be sure to eat about 20 to 30 percent of your daily food intake as fat.

Aside from this list of benefits, fats also help satisfy your hunger because they take longer to empty from the stomach than other foods. And, let's not forget that fats carry the flavor of food and feel satisfying in the mouth.

> **Lean Lingo**
>
> **Insulin** is a hormone secreted by the pancreas gland. It regulates the level of sugar (glucose) in the blood and one of the hormones that causes the body to store fat. **Dietary fats** are fats you eat. Body fat refers to the fat your body stores in the adipose tissues of your body. Your body can produce body fat from dietary fats, carbohydrates, or proteins.

Types of Fats

Fats are the most highly concentrated form of fuel. They contain more calories per ounce than either proteins or carbs. Fats come in three basic forms: saturated, polyunsaturated, and monounsaturated. Plus, today there's a fourth type of artificial fat present in food called trans fats. It can contribute to heart disease, so avoid eating trans fats.

The degree of saturation of a fat refers to its arrangement of carbon and hydrogen atoms. A saturated fat is one that carries the maximum number of hydrogen atoms in its carbon chain. It's "saturated." An unsaturated fat has room for additional hydrogen atoms, which tends to make it more biologically active.

Saturated Fats

Saturated fats come mostly from animal products, including milk and milk products, and from several vegetables:

Butter	Milk
Cheese	Beef
Lamb	Veal
Pork	Poultry
Lard	Vegetable shortening
Cocoa butter	Palm oil
Coconut oil	Kernel oil

Limit your intake of saturated fat to no more than 10 percent of your food intake daily. So, yes, enjoy your beef and butter, but in moderation.

Polyunsaturated Fats

Polyunsaturated fats are found in seeds, seed oils, and vegetable oils, as well as in cold-water fish. The following are common sources of polyunsaturated fats:

Corn oil	Safflower oil
Sunflower oil	Soybean oil
Flaxseed oil	Salmon
Mackerel	Herring
Cod	Sardines
Albacore tuna	Black currants
Flaxseeds	Sunflower seeds
Corn	Evening primrose

Monounsaturated Fats

Monounsaturated fats are found in certain vegetable oils and nut oils, which are best when unprocessed. The following are common sources of monounsaturated fats:

Olive oil	Sesame Seeds
Canola oil	Sesame seed oil
Peanuts	Almonds
Peanut oil	Almond oil
Avocados	

Trans Fats

Trans fats are man-made fats created by transforming unsaturated fats into saturated fats through heat and hydrogenation (adding hydrogen atoms). They're also called "partially hydrogenated" oils. Once a favorite of the food industry, studies show that trans fats harm your health and can directly cause heart disease, as well as increased insulin production, decreased testosterone, lower metabolism, and raise bad cholesterol levels. The FDA now requires that food labels state the amount of trans fats per serving. It's best to avoid them.

Yes, Fats Are Also Essential

Just as we noted that your body needs essential amino acids for good health, so, too, does your body require *essential fatty acids (EFAs)*. Your body can't synthesize these from other foods you eat. You must ingest them.

EFAs are beneficial for hormone production. The brain needs EFAs to function properly, and they are critical for the transmission of nerve impulses. EFAs also aid you in many other ways. They help ...

Lean Lingo

Your body needs **essential fatty acids (EFAs)** for important metabolic processes. EFAs are fats that cannot be synthesized by your body; they must be ingested.

   ◆ Regulate the transport of oxygen and energy through your body.

   ◆ Form new cells, particularly in the nervous system.

   ◆ Increase your body's metabolic rate.

   ◆ Improve skin and hair.

   ◆ Help reduce high blood pressure.

   ◆ Help lower cholesterol and triglyceride levels.

As you can see, you need your EFAs. There are two kinds of essential fatty acids that are derived from fat sources containing the omega-3 and omega-6 fatty acids.

Omega-3s

Omega-3s consist of docosahexaenoic, eicosapentaenoic, and alpha-linolenic acids. The first two are considered to be the most important omega-3s and are found only in deep-water fish like salmon. Alpha-linolenic acid is found in deep-water fish, emu, fish oil, and some vegetable-based oils, including flaxseed and walnut oil.

Omega-3s have become less common in the American diet over the past 50 years ... which is unfortunate. They offer powerful health and weight-loss benefits. They help rev up your fat-burning mechanism. Because they're harder to find in today's modern foods, we recommend that you take omega-3s in a nutritional supplement, such as fish oil. These fats are quite beneficial because they have an anti-inflammatory effect on the body.

Omega-6s

Omega-6 fatty acids consist of linoleic and gamma-linolenic acids. They are found in raw nuts, seeds, and legumes and in such unsaturated oils as borage, grape seed, primrose, sesame, and olive oil. The omega-6 fatty acids in these oils are destroyed when heated, so they should be consumed in an uncooked and unprocessed form. You eat plenty of these in processed foods. Eating too many processed foods that contain omega-6s can cause inflammation.

How Much Fat Is Too Much Fat?

Studies show that the average American diet consists of about 39 percent fat. Wow! That is more than enough. The American Heart Association suggests we keep our fat intake to 30 percent or less.

Limit saturated fats to 10 percent of your total food intake, with the rest of your fat intake coming from monounsaturated and polyunsaturated fats. Consume at least 10 percent, preferably 20 percent, of your total calories from food sources or supplements with EFAs.

Stay away from most low-fat processed foods. Search them out in your house and toss them. True, they're low in fat, but they simply can't deliver on the implied promise of a lean trim body.

Fat Shopping and Eating Tips

The following is a list of good fats to buy at the store:

◆ **Olive oil.** The darker the better because it's the least refined or processed and has the most good-for-you oils.

◆ **Butter.** Yes, butter is fine to eat in small amounts. Good for sautéing and baking because it doesn't break down into trans fats, like vegetable oils do.

◆ **Salmon.** It's rich in omega-3 EFAs and polyunsaturated fats. Poach or bake more than enough for dinner so that you can enjoy salmon salad—made with real mayonnaise—the next day.

◆ **Other cold-water fish.** These include mackerel, albacore tuna, sardines, and lake trout.

◆ **Real versions of anything you have eaten as a low-fat processed food.** We're talking about real ice cream, real salad dressing, real butter, real mayonnaise, and so on.

◆ **Canola oil.** Also considered a monounsaturated fat, it is an alternative to olive oil for salads.

◆ **Nuts and seeds.** Great for snacks, but eat in small quantities.

◆ **Fish oil from the health-food store.** This comes in bottles and is refrigerated. Use as a dietary supplement.

◆ **Avocados and olives.** These contain monounsaturated fats and add great flavor to meals.

Use olive oil and other cold-expeller pressed oils for salads; use butter for sautéing. And enjoy nuts, seeds, avocados, and olives as snacks and as condiments for salads and main dishes.

Thinspiration

If you want the healthiest salad dressing when eating at a restaurant, ask for olive oil and vinegar. The olive oil is a monounsaturated oil. If you prefer more flavor, ask for some crumbled blue cheese to go with it.

Carbohydrates

When many people talk about carbohydrates, they're usually talking about starches and sugars. But carbohydrates are more than that. They include starches such as bread and potatoes, as well as sugars, fruits, vegetables, and of course, a common favorite, chocolate. Here's your chance to get a better understanding of how to eat carbs wisely.

Carbs Are for Energy

Almost all carbohydrates come to us from plants. The only animal products that contain carbohydrates are milk and milk products. Most people—and especially people who are overweight—love carbs, especially starchy cakes, cookies, pastas, and bagels. We call these the fluffy starches. Yes, they're fattening. Eat too many carbs, and your body turns them into fatty acids and stores them as fat.

Your brain, with its many complex chemical reactions, gets a mild tranquilizing effect when you eat carbs. Carbs lift your serotonin levels. You have experienced this effect if you have ever used carbs to soothe anxiety, nerves, or a low emotional feeling.

Most unprocessed carbohydrates contain fiber. The less processed the carb, the higher the fiber content. Fiber aids your digestion because it retains water and adds bulk, thus helping with proper elimination. High-fiber diets have been shown to help lower cholesterol levels because the fiber absorbs fat, thus lowering fat levels, and reduce the incidence of colon cancer by absorbing toxins and moving them quickly through the digestive system and out of the body.

Carbs, Insulin, and Your Weight

Not all carbohydrates are created equal. Some definitely are better for you than others. That's because different carbohydrates affect blood sugar levels differently. The blood sugar level, or glucose level in the bloodstream, is our primary source of energy. We simply can't live without a sufficient amount. But if there ever was a perfect example of "too much of a good thing," blood sugar is it. When you eat a carbohydrate, it lifts your blood sugar. Then the pancreas secrets a hormone called *insulin*. Insulin keeps your blood sugar in the safe range. So far, so good. You eat some carbs, your blood sugar rises, your pancreas secretes insulin, and your blood sugar level returns to normal. This happens every time you eat carbohydrates. This is normal.

When someone continually has high blood sugar, the body's cells become insensitive to insulin, and blood sugar can't leave the bloodstream. Someone with a fasting (meaning the person hasn't eaten for 12 hours or more) blood sugar level of 126 or above is used as a diagnostic indicator of type 2 diabetes. Normal, healthy blood-sugar levels range between 70 and 110. The guidelines measure milligrams of glucose per one tenth liter of blood.

Herein lies the rub. Some carbohydrates cause blood sugar levels to jump higher than others. This causes the pancreas to secrete more insulin to stabilize the blood sugar. Because of the spike in blood sugar, the pancreas in a sense overreacts and puts out lots of insulin. After your blood sugar stabilizes, extra insulin can be hanging around in your blood stream.

What are the consequences of excess insulin in your bloodstream?

1. **It makes you hungry again right away.** Think of when you start the day with a donut. Soon after eating it you feel hungry again, so you eat one or two more. Pretty soon the box is empty. The excess insulin in your blood stream gave you a sense of false hunger.

2. **It stores fat.** Yes, excess insulin causes the body to store more body fat. You could be on a low-calorie diet and still be storing fat because you're eating quick-acting carbohydrates. Ah-ha, you might be saying, that explains it!

Ideally, you should avoid eating quick-acting carbs and instead dine on the ones that don't trigger a fast insulin response. Many overweight people finally begin to master their weight when they learn how to manage their carb intake.

The Carbohydrate Hit List

So what carbs are the "thinnest?" First in Australia, then in Canada, and finally in the United States, researchers and dietitians are using a concept called glycemic indexing. The index is a measure of the blood sugar response of various carbs.

The researchers tested subjects—people like you and me—by having them eat plain old white bread. The researchers then measured the test subjects' blood sugar responses to get a baseline. They assigned white bread the value of 100. They subsequently fed the test subjects virtually all known carbohydrates at separate times. For each food, they measured the blood sugar of the subjects. The result was the glycemic index. The research has been compiled into glycemic index lists, now available via the

Internet and in various books. A value of 14, peanuts, is lowest. Highest is 115 for frozen tofu dessert. Refer to Appendix B for how to obtain the Glycemic Index.

Understanding and Using the Glycemic Index

Foods that have a glycemic index score of 70 or higher are considered high-glycemic, foods scoring in the 40 to 69 range are considered moderate-glycemic, and foods scoring 39 and below are considered low-glycemic.

The following is an overview of glycemic indexing that is simple and easy to remember. That way, you don't need to keep a chart in your wallet to eat with confidence.

Here is our ranking of carbohydrates, from worst to best:

1. **Starches.** These include processed wheat products, white potatoes, and all foods made from them: bagels, pasta, cookies, cake, muffins, chips, crackers, popcorn, baked potatoes, rice cakes, and such. Remember eating rice cakes, thinking they didn't have many calories? They don't, but they are ranked as one of the highest foods for stimulating blood sugar (at 82). Oh, dear.

2. **Sugars.** These include table sugar and most candy. Also honey, molasses, and rice syrup. Sugars are moderate- to high-glycemic. When reading the label, an ingredient ending in "-ose" indicates a sugar. The glycemic index is about 68.

3. **Chocolate.** We just had to give chocolate its own listing. We know you desperately want to know whether you should give up your chocolate. Chocolate is low-glycemic. Dark chocolate is about 48. Milk chocolate and white chocolate are higher because they contain more sugar, but they are still low-glycemic. What makes chocolate low-glycemic is the fat content.

4. **Fruits.** These include most fruits such as apples, grapes, oranges, strawberries, cantaloupe, figs, berries, and pears. Fruits are mostly low-glycemic or moderate-glycemic. The glycemic index range is typically 0–50.

5. **Vegetables.** These include most vegetables except for some higher-glycemic types like many types of white potatoes, parsnips, and pumpkin. Vegetables that are low-glycemic have a glycemic index range from about 0 to 64.

In summary, fluffy white starches raise blood sugar levels the fastest and the highest, followed by sugars, chocolate, fruits, and vegetables, the lowest blood sugar stimulators.

Eating Carbs with Confidence

Yes, you can still enjoy your favorite carbohydrate treats. As part of your overall food consumption, carbs should be about 35 to 50 percent of your caloric intake. Eat fewer of the high-glycemic carbs, and instead eat the low-glycemic carbs.

Sugar Is Sweet and Okay to Eat ... Sometimes

Some sugars, such as table sugar or sucrose, are one notch below starches on the glycemic index because they stimulate blood sugar slower than many of the starches (the fluffy whites). It's okay to have some sugar. Really. A spoonful of sugar in tea or coffee is fine, but a bagful of candy is too much. You knew this already because a whole bag would take you way beyond 5 on the hunger scale.

Most of the time, when people say they are hooked on sugar, they really mean they are hooked on starches that contain sugars. Very few people eat sugar directly from the bowl. Take away the starch part of the cookie and not much is left.

Fruit Is Yummy

We are now at the place in the glycemic list where you can relax. Fruits are terrific for you. Enjoy them. The new dietary guidelines recommend eating five to ten servings of fresh fruits and vegetables a day. So go for it. Enjoy an orange for breakfast and berries for dinner.

All fruits contain vital *nutrients* and important sugars that your body needs for health. Fruits also are abundant in fiber, which is important for good health and timely elimination.

Veggies for You and Me

You can't go wrong eating vegetables. Think salads (more on salad dressing in the next chapter on fats), broccoli, spinach, and snow peas. Remember cauliflower, celery, green beans, zucchini, summer squash, and cabbage. And don't forget tomatoes, cucumbers, and radishes. The list goes on and on.

Vegetables are positively packed with health-giving nutrients. They contain lots of fiber plus phytonutrients that protect us from disease and aid our immune functioning. They contain a wealth of antioxidants to neutralize cell damage that happens in our everyday life.

If the glycemic index seems more complicated than you want, consider this: Your stomach is only about the size of your fist when unstretched, give or take. In a meal containing protein, carbohydrates, and fats, only 40 to 55 percent of the calories in that fist-size collection of food should be your carbohydrates. Since your carbohydrate intake should include five servings of fresh fruits and vegetables a day, just how much room is left for starches and sugars? That's right, about a condiment size.

> **Lean Lingo**
>
> **Nutrient density** describes the extent to which a food supplies all kinds of nutrients— vitamins, minerals, phytonutrients, antioxidants, enzymes, and energy. **Glycemic load** is a calculation that indicates the impact of total carbohydrates eaten on a person's blood sugar level. Aim for eating 75 to 100 glycemic load units a day, with about 25–30 at each meal.

Nutrient-Rich Foods

Here's how to get the most nutrients from that modest amount of food that fits into the size of your fist. Dietitians call it *nutrient density*. The idea of nutrient density is to get as many nutrients as possible in the food you eat. For example, if you want a sweet-tasting liquid, you get more nutrients from the same amount of orange juice as from a soft drink or soda. You get more nutrients from an apple than from a slice of white bread. You get more nutrients from barley pilaf than from white rice, even if it is enriched rice. You certainly get more nutrients from a green salad than from potato chips.

But What about My Treats?

When you want a treat, plan for it in your day's eating. That way, it's included in eating 0–5, and it's budgeted into your total carbohydrate intake. Sound challenging or nearly impossible? If you follow eating 0–5 closely and eat nutrient-dense foods about 80 to 90 percent of the time, you can have a treat every day. Remember to factor it into the 35 to 50 percent of your total carbohydrate eating.

Another way to look at treats is that rather than going for volume, go for quality and eat only the best. Then eat sensuously. So, if you want a treat after dinner, and you haven't reached a 5 on the hunger scale, you can have your treat. Just make sure that you don't eat above 5. The treat can be what you want—chocolate chips, a bite or two of cheesecake, whatever.

Carbohydrate Loading Is Too Big a Load

Yes, that "too much of a good thing" adage applies to even low-glycemic foods. There's always the temptation to "carbohydrate load," that is, eating too many low-glycemic foods. When you do, the high quantity of carbohydrate causes the blood sugar to spike and then the pancreas reacts as if a person ate a smaller amount of a high-glycemic food, pumping more insulin into the bloodstream than necessary. The excess insulin causes the body to store fat. So, too, many low-glycemic carbs can also cause the body to store fat. Some semolina spaghetti is low-glycemic, but going back for a second serving could make it high-glycemic.

Another way to carbohydrate load is to have too many types of carbohydrates in one meal. For example, semolina spaghetti with tomato and vegetable sauce, a salad with croutons, steamed carrots, and a cookie for dessert would constitute carbohydrate loading. So, too, would a meal of tofu, rice, beans, bread, and pie for dessert. Although each of these items would be acceptable as part of a regular meal, the combination makes your *glycemic load* too high.

Even when you eat from 0–5, avoid carbohydrate loading if you want to get your best weight-loss results.

The Least You Need to Know

- Glycemic indexing rates carbohydrates by how they raise blood sugar, which can cause the body to store fat. Carbohydrates include starches, sugars, fruits, and vegetables.

- Dietary fat is essential for your well-being and attaining your ideal size; eating the right dietary fats enables your body to release fat.

- By eating adequate protein, your body obtains the building blocks of life, the essential amino acids.

- Protein gives you energy, staves off fatigue, and helps regulate blood sugar.

Other Foods We Eat

In This Chapter

- ◆ Artificial foods you could eat
- ◆ What artificial foods do for weight loss
- ◆ Eating fewer fake foods

When is a food not a food? Only carbohydrates, proteins, and fats are natural energy food sources. But in our modern world, you also ingest many other things that don't fall into these three categories.

You need to know which things definitely to include in your eating, which ones to avoid, and which ones to use with care.

Nonfood No-No's

You eat plenty of substances that haven't the faintest resemblance to food. Sometimes you eat them because they are hidden in foods, especially processed foods. Sometimes you eat them because you think they will help you lose weight. Some of them are good for weight loss; some are bad; and some are neutral.

Additives and artificial ingredients are typically added to foods in very small amounts, but the average American consumes an estimated five pounds of additives each year. Wow! That's a lot of chemicals. The sections that follow have the rundown on such substances.

Preservatives, Flavorings, and Food Dyes

These substances are man-made, engineered to preserve the grocery shelf life of processed foods, to enhance flavor, or to give coloring. Most of the time, they are the unpronounceable words on the food label. They aren't nutritive; in other words, your body won't use them for energy or health. In fact, while some of them are considered safe by FDA standards, they might not be good for you or your weight-loss program.

Thinspiration

As best as you can, eat unrefined and unprocessed foods, such as meats, vegetables, and fruits. Your body knows how to digest these. As dietary staples, they are the key to life-long weight maintenance.

Try to eliminate or cut back on processed foods in your diet. We realize this isn't always easy. Because of our busy lives, we have grown accustomed to eating prepared foods that are ready to be popped into the microwave. However, your overall nutrition will improve, as will your weight loss, if you orient your diet to natural foods—protein, carbs, and fats—and eliminate these additives.

One of our clients, Anita, loves ice cream. As part of her program to manage her eating and her weight, she went grocery shopping to buy natural ice cream. Brand after brand contained unnatural mystery ingredients. She said her hands got quite cold before she finally found a carton that contained pure food ingredients, such as cream, eggs, sugar, and milk. But it sure tasted good, and it was better for her family.

This brings us to another reason for turning up your nose at these artificial ingredients, which we not-so-affectionately refer to as "mystery" ingredients. These include such chemicals as sodium nitrite, BHA, sulfur dioxide, sodium sulfite, calcium disodium EDTA, polysorbate 60, calcium propionate, potassium sorbate, ammonium sulfate, sodium propionate, and disodium inosinate. Also included are colors with numbers, such as yellow 5 or 6. The body doesn't know what to make of these chemicals.

We all hope or assume that our bodies will simply excrete them and let them pass on through without doing us any bodily harm, but experts now think that the body treats such foreign substances as toxins. The ones that aren't excreted are stored in body fat. Recent studies suggest that a person's body might create even more body fat so that it has more room to store the onslaught of toxins. This means that some of your weight gain could be intentional—you body needs more fat in order to store all the toxins you eat.

A smart strategy is to "just say no" to artificial anything in your food as best as you can.

Artificial Sweeteners

Pass on artificial sweeteners, too. Try to eliminate aspartame, sucralose, and saccharine from your diet. They are nonnutritive. Ask yourself how many pounds you have lost since you started drinking diet sodas. Are they working? Most likely not. Here's why.

Recent studies suggest that artificial sweeteners boost your insulin levels by fooling the body into reacting to them as it does to sugar. This is bad for weight loss and maintenance. The more insulin in your bloodstream, the more fat your body stores. If you are hooked on either aspartame or saccharine, it not only can be detrimental to your health, it also can stall and thwart your weight-loss progress. Give up artificial sweeteners.

CAUTION

Weighty Warning

The Food and Drug Administration (FDA) has received reports of aspartame being linked to seizures, visual impairment, pancreas inflammation, and high blood pressure, among other disorders. The warning label on saccharine states that consumption is linked to cancer. These artificial sweeteners, as well as monosodium glutamate (MSG), are called "excitotoxins" because they affect the brain negatively.

Another sugar substitute is called sucralose, with the brand name of Splenda. We don't recommend it because it's manufactured by adding chlorine molecules to regular sugar. One of the reasons we recommend drinking purified water is to avoid drinking the chlorine. So to consume sucralose and put unnecessary chlorine back in the body makes no sense. Sucralose contains high-glycemic starches as a filler, and no one needs them either.

Other beverages you can substitute for diet sodas and other beverages sweetened with aspartame, sucralose, or saccharin are herbal teas, decaffeinated coffee, or purified water. Try flavoring purified water with lemon or lime juice.

Healthy and Natural Sugar Substitutes

You don't need to live a life without the wonderful taste of sweetness. Nature has given us plenty of choices. Choose from these to sweeten your coffee or tea. They can even work well for baked goods.

 ◆ Stevia with FOS. Stevia is a very sweet herb from South America that's available in powder and liquid form at health-food stores. FOS stands for fruit ogiliosac-charides, which are beneficial for and support healthy intestinal bacteria, or flora. Stevia with FOS is a nonnutritive powder found at health-food stores or in the health-food section of your grocery store. Be careful—a little goes a long way.

 ◆ Single blossom honey, such as red clover honey, or orange blossom honey is low-glycemic. You can comfortably use this to sweeten your beverages. The same with Agave nectar. Both, however, are high-caloric and high-carbohydrate, so use sparingly.

 ◆ Xylitol, known as birch sugar, can be used for baking and sweetening beverages. Xylitol is low-glycemic and healthy for you. It doesn't cause blood sugar imbalances or yeast overgrowth like table sugar. It's thought to promote bone health and prevent tooth decay and plaque buildup. The only drawback is that if you eat too much, you could experience gastrointestinal discomfort and diarrhea. But then, if you're eating 0–5, you won't be eating too much.

 ◆ Fructose is a natural low-glycemic sugar that's found in fruit. You can also find it in granulated form at health-food stores. Fructose is sweeter than regular table sugar, so you need less. Research indicates that ingesting lots of fructose, as in drinking sodas and beverages sweetened with high-fructose corn syrup, and using processed foods, such as syrups and candy that contain high-fructose corn syrup, can elevate the lipids that increase heart disease. So stay away from those syrupy and sweet processed foods. But you're fine eating fruit and using fructose sparingly as a sweetener and for baking.

 ◆ Sucrose, or regular table sugar, is medium-glycemic and fine for most people if you consume small amounts, as in sweetening your coffee. Eating large amounts, for instance, in candy and baked goods, isn't on your eating plan, and eating large amounts of anything will ruin your 0–5 eating.

You can use natural sweeteners with confidence, but of course, with restraint.

MSG

Monosodium glutamate (MSG) is used as a flavor enhancer. It actually gives your tongue's taste buds for protein a false positive indication. The glutamine in MSG is what your taste buds sense and tells you that you're eating protein. Of course, the MSG fools you. It isn't protein, but it is added to many foods, especially soups, stews, and meat-free foods, to intensify the protein taste and to fool your body into sensing that the food has far more animal protein than it actually has.

MSG is renowned for causing headaches and other undesirable side effects. Avoid MSG when you can. At Asian restaurants, where MSG usage is common practice, ask for your food to be prepared without MSG. Check food labels for the presence of MSG. Its effect on actual weight gain or loss is unknown, but it certainly doesn't promote health.

Weighty Warning

Read the labels carefully if you want to avoid monosodium glutamate. Look for these other terms for MSG: meat tenderizer, hydrolyzed protein, textured protein, hydrolyzed oat flour, calcium caseinate, sodium caseinate, autolyzed yeast, and yeast extract. MSG is commonly found in fast foods, dairy products, salad dressings, nondairy creamers, sausage and bacon, lunchmeats, canned soups and sauces, cocoa mixes, and veggie burgers.

Alcoholic Beverages

Alcohol isn't exactly a weight-loss no-no, but we can't fully endorse it, so we include it in this section. Including alcohol in your weight-loss plan requires care and forethought. Because alcohol isn't a protein, fat, or carbohydrate, we don't classify it as a food. In fact, our wonderful internal food processor and detoxifier, the liver, treats alcohol as a poison.

As for weight loss, well, alcohol is tricky. You need to treat it as a food because alcohol changes your hunger numbers. Alcoholic drinks also contain calories. Your body metabolizes alcohol into sugar. What isn't used for energy is converted into fat. Be sure to account for it in your total food intake.

Alcohol is cortisol-stimulating. When you have a drink, your body's levels of this stress hormone rise. High cortisol levels cause the body to store fat, specifically around the abdomen and waist. One key to weight loss is to keep your cortisol levels low.

Alcohol is an appetite stimulant. It can stimulate you to eat more food than you need (that is, to eat above a 5 on the hunger scale). Alcohol is also a depressant, so it can dull your ability to feel your hunger numbers. This means that you could overeat because you couldn't feel your stomach hunger sensations.

Alcohol affects each person quite differently. We know one woman who lost seven sizes, from a size 22 to a size 8, and still drank a glass of wine with dinner every night. Find out how it affects you. If you suspect that alcohol is interfering with your weight loss, stop consuming it.

Yes, Have Water

Drinking water is essential for weight loss. Purified water is best. Have a minimum of eight glasses of water a day, more if you are thirsty or when you are exercising. A handy rule of thumb is to have as many ounces of water as your weight in pounds divided by two. If you weigh about 150, you require 75 ounces of water per day, or about nine 8-ounce glasses. No acceptable substitutes for water exist. Herbal teas, coffee, sodas, and other liquids are not the same as water.

Water constitutes roughly 70 percent of your body and is involved in digestion, absorption, circulation, and excretion. It is critical to the transport of waste products out of your body resulting from your digestion and metabolic processes. As you release excess fat, the toxins stored in body fat are released into your body. Water is essential to flush out these toxins and the toxins hanging around in your bladder, liver, kidney, and bloodstream. How much more motivation do you need?

Don't wait until you are thirsty to drink water. When you wait that long, you are already dehydrated. Dehydration can confuse the hunger/thirst mechanism in the brain, making you think you are hungry when in fact you aren't. If you drink water regularly throughout the day, it will boost your energy, help satisfy your "mouth hunger," and decrease the likelihood that you will experience headaches, muscle aches, food allergies, or acid stomach.

If you find it a challenge to drink enough water, we recommend that you get in the habit of drinking four to eight ounces every hour on the hour. Just do it. The body will absorb smaller amounts like this more easily and will not excrete it as fast—so you'll make fewer trips to the bathroom versus drinking 16 ounces or more at a time!

We recommend that you take a water bottle with you when you are out and about—running errands or attending your kids' soccer games. Sipping on water keeps your energy level higher and allows for clearer thinking.

Can you drink too much water? One dieter e-mailed that she was drinking 30 glasses of water a day! She wanted to know why she hadn't lost any weight. She probably knew the locations of every public restroom within a 100-mile radius of her home, but this huge amount of water wasn't helping her. While we applaud drinking water, it alone can't make you lose weight. Without enough water, however, you will likely inhibit your ability to lose weight. For more about water and hydration, read the "Electrolytes" section in Chapter 11.

> **CAUTION**
> **Weighty Warning**
> You have an increased chance of being chronically dehydrated if you are obese (BMI over 30). This is because the body actually has a lower water percentage the higher your body-fat percentage is. You will have more difficulty releasing weight because you are dehydrated. Hydrating your body will help you release fat.

Drinking Quality Water

By drinking purified water, you reduce your exposure to certain environmental toxins found in tap water, such as chlorine, pesticides, other chemicals, and parasites. Tap water has been shown to contain chemicals from perfumes, prescription medications, caffeine, industrial runoff, and agricultural production.

Tap water purity standards vary from one water district to another. You might want to ask your public water company for its water-quality report to see what you are drinking. For instance, arsenic concentrations vary quite a lot from one part of the country to the next.

Reduce any possible risk to your health by drinking purified water. You can purchase artesian water or purified water at the store, install a water purifier under your kitchen sink or attach one to the main water supply in your house. Because distilled water is devoid of all nutrients, including valuable trace minerals, we don't recommend drinking it.

The Least You Need To Know

◆ Avoid eating artificial foods, such as preservatives, flavorings, and colorings; replace artificial sweeteners with Stevia with FOS or single blossom honey.

◆ The toxins in artificial foods are stored in body fat, so avoid eating them when you can to reduce your body burden.

◆ Drink at least eight glasses of purified water every day to keep your body hydrated and facilitate weight loss.

Chapter 11

Supplementation

In This Chapter

- Taking supplements for weight-loss support
- What supplements can and can't do
- Product claims versus reality

Taking dietary supplements is fast becoming an American way of life. The medical profession now advises taking multivitamins, and new research is published weekly about the health benefits of phytonutrients, antioxidants, and other micronutrients available in foods and supplemental form.

Most likely you've acquired various bottles and jars of supplements to enhance your weight loss. In this chapter, we help you sift through the hype to learn which supplements can aid you in weight loss and which ones won't make much difference. Oh yes, and which ones are potentially harmful or are simply a waste of money.

Supplements as Support, Not Cure-All

You're probably aware of—in fact, you probably feel bombarded by— health claims for certain supplements. TV infomercials, radio stations, newspapers, and magazines are bursting with magical claims for various pills and potions. Kind of confusing and intimidating, isn't it?

Lean Lingo _____

Vitamins and minerals often are referred to as **micronutrients** because your body needs only tiny amounts compared to the four basic nutrients: protein, fats, carbohydrates, and water.

The supplements category includes _micronutrients—_ vitamins and minerals—as well as protein supplements, oils, and metabolic boosters.

Although we doubt anyone has ever lost weight just by taking certain vitamins and minerals, your body needs more nutritional support while you are losing weight. In a sense, losing weight stresses the body. Yes, losing weight is good for your overall health and well-being, but the very activity of releasing fat causes internal stress of its own.

Because your stored fat holds toxins—that's where the body stores them—when you start losing weight, the toxins are released from the fat to be processed by your liver and excreted. This takes extra work. When releasing fat, some people report feeling sort of "yucky" for weeks or months as the toxin load in their vital organs increases.

Think of nutritional supplements as insurance. If you're eating healthy meals including cold-water fish for essential fatty acids two or three times a week and five to ten daily servings of vegetables and fruit, you may already be ingesting adequate amounts of vitamins, minerals, antioxidants, and EFAs. But just because you ingest them doesn't mean that your body digests and assimilates them well. In which case, supplements are your insurance. Ditto if you don't always eat healthy meals.

With the right kinds of supplementation, you can decrease the toxin load and feel more energized as the fat flushes out. You might also notice that some of your food cravings diminish or simply go away when you take certain supplements. They can increase your stamina and overall energy level as you get to your ideal size.

Antioxidants

Hooray for antioxidants! The various metabolic processes that break down stored fat molecules release _free radicals_ such as superoxide radicals, hydroxyl radicals, hypochlorite radicals, hydrogen peroxide, various lipid peroxides, and nitric acid. Free radicals can be quite damaging to your health. They've been closely linked to cancer and other serious illnesses.

Eating fruits and vegetables gives you antioxidants that help your body neutralize the free radicals being released in your body while you're shedding excess fat. The support you get from antioxidants helps you feel better during your weight-loss process.

Certain phytochemicals in your diet also act as antioxidants that neutralize free radicals or support body functions that do. These include vitamins A, C, and E, beta-carotene, flavonoids, and the mineral selenium. These antioxidants are abundant in the five or more daily servings of fresh fruits and vegetables that you're eating, and some are in the essential fatty acids (EFAs). You can also obtain these antioxidants through supplements.

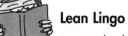

Lean Lingo

Free radicals are unstable, hyperactive molecules that damage healthy cells and tissues.

Vitamins

Vitamins are required for the many metabolic processes that release the energy from the food you digest. Right now, as you are losing weight, you want the most energy possible from your food. B vitamins work together synergistically to boost metabolism, maintain healthy skin and muscle tone, enhance immune functions, and promote healthy cells. Several of the B vitamins are critical to the conversion of fats, carbs, and proteins into energy. You need a nutritional boost during this time of physical and emotional changes, so take a multivitamin and mineral supplement that supplies a balanced formulation.

Look for the tagline, "bio-available," when shopping for supplements. This means the product is formulated to be readily digested and assimilated in your body. Some supplements are hard to digest and have a molecular structure that isn't easily used by your body. You can find high-quality vitamin and mineral supplements at your health-food store and online.

B Vitamins for Stress

When you're under stress, your body quickly uses up its B vitamins. Because B vitamins are water-soluble, what you don't use in a day or so is eliminated from your body. This means you need a daily dose of Bs.

How do you get vitamin Bs? All meats—especially organ meats, such as liver—contain high concentrations of B vitamins. Next best are fruits and vegetables, especially green leafy vegetables. (You're eating those regularly now, right?) Fish, poultry, eggs, and dairy products also contain some of the different B vitamins. Still, your stressed-out body might not be receiving enough of these stress-fighting vitamins.

Unfortunately, B vitamins are also the hardest to digest and assimilate. They require a fully functioning digestive system every step of the way. If your stomach doesn't secrete enough intrinsic factor, a chemical substance produced by the stomach, you won't be able to absorb B-12. This condition can be remedied by taking liquid or sublingual B-12 formulations. These liquids or dissolving tablets bypass the stomach and are instead absorbed in the mucous lining of the mouth. If you don't have adequate lactobacillus bacteria in the large intestine, you won't process and assimilate all the B vitamins you need. This can sometimes be remedied by taking a lactobacillus supplement.

B vitamins are included in most multivitamin supplements at your health-food store. Get your B vitamins from as many sources as you can—meat, fruits, veggies, fish, poultry, eggs, or supplements—and get them every day. Take more if you have a high stress load.

Minerals

You need minerals for the maintenance of healthy nerves, tissues, muscle, and bones. You also need them for proper muscle functioning and high metabolism. Chromium, for instance, works with insulin to regulate the body's use of sugars and fatty acid metabolism. Minerals play a role in proper hydration. If your minerals are way out of balance, you could be drinking all the glasses of water available in the world and still not be hydrated.

There are two types of minerals that your body needs:

1. **Macrominerals** are needed in large amounts. These include calcium, magnesium, sodium, chloride, potassium, and phosphorus. These are in the foods you eat. You also can get them in most multivitamin and mineral supplements. These minerals are essential for you to have the proper electrolyte balance in your body.

2. **Microminerals** are needed in very small amounts in your body. Even though you need only trace amounts—that's why they're often called "trace elements"— they are required for good health and for mental and emotional stability. Microminerals include chromium, iron, iodine, copper, cesium, lithium, platinum, selenium, vanadium, zinc, manganese, and boron. Altogether your body needs more than 70 trace elements. You can get them from animal protein and from your five servings of fruits and vegetables. When you are losing weight, be sure to get enough but not too much. To assure that you ingest enough of these micronutrients, consider taking a trace mineral supplement. See Appendix B for supplement suggestions.

Although all of the minerals listed here are essential for your health, two additional minerals should be noted for aiding in weight loss:

◆ **Calcium.** Take a calcium supplement daily that contains about 500 to 1500 mg. Research shows that women who take extra calcium can lose more weight and keep it off more easily. It's best to obtain your calcium from a supplement that contains bio-available calcium. Also, calcium can be ingested by eating foods such as dark green leafy vegetables, sardines, salmon canned with bones, oysters, broccoli, some legumes such as kidney beans and great northern beans, blackstrap molasses, and dairy products. Don't rely on dairy products for adequate calcium—one tablespoon of blackstrap molasses provides more calcium than a full glass of milk.

> **CAUTION**
>
> **Weighty Warning**
>
> A hundred years ago, it was easier to get the minerals you needed from food. But growing soils have become more depleted in the age of agribusiness. Today, we cannot be sure that our grocery-store produce was grown in mineral-rich soil.

◆ **Chromium.** Chromium helps your body retain lean muscle mass while you're losing weight, so that you lose more fat than muscle. Chromium also stabilizes blood sugar levels, helping you avoid frantic overeating if your blood sugar level drops throughout the day. Taking 400 to 600 mcg a day can reduce insulin resistance and assist with weight loss. Food sources that are high in chromium include brewers yeast, dairy products, wheat germ, oats, meat, chicken, and fish.

Electrolytes

You must have the proper electrolyte balance in your body to get all the value from the water you drink. Jane, in her 30s, was constantly thirsty and drank water all day long. She carried a water bottle with her wherever she went. When she had her body-fat percentage measured, she was startled to learn that she was dehydrated! How could that be? Jane's electrolytes were out of balance. Basically, no amount of water was going to get her fully re-hydrated.

You obtain electrolytes from your food, but it's possible to be depleted from sweating due to exercise, exposure to heat from the sun or saunas, or health conditions such as vomiting or diarrhea.

Sports drinks contain electrolytes, but many come with a price tag of high-glycemic sugars such as high-fructose corn syrup. You don't want to drink a beverage for electrolytes and in the process trigger an overload of insulin that stores fat. That wouldn't help much. Avoid sports drinks, which are typically high-glycemic. Instead, mix a packet of Emergen-C, which is available in health-food stores, in water. See Appendix B for more specific recommendations.

If It's Green, It's Good

Many people who struggle to lose weight have recurrent yeast overgrowth problems. If you're a woman, you know whether you have the obvious vaginal yeast infection. But you can have yeast infections in your bowels, ears, and plenty of other places in your body. Many people struggle with these for years. Some go on the recommended yeast-free diets for years and still have yeast overgrowth. Many take prescription medications continually.

When a person can eliminate yeast overgrowth syndrome it's easier to lose weight. Our clients have experienced terrific success by drinking greens formulations. These powders are filled with good-for-you green things such as chlorella, spirulina, barley grass, wheat grass, and other nutrients. In addition to supplying phytonutrients, antioxidants, and vitamins, the drinks make the body slightly alkaline. Since yeast grows best in an acidic body environment, the alkalinity helps kill off the yeast, freeing you up to lose weight.

Thinspiration

One client baked bread every day and was continually exposed to yeast spores. She had yeast growth throughout her body and on her skin. She didn't want to stop baking bread because it was an activity she did with her husband. So she started taking a greens drink and within a couple of weeks had lost a dress size. Her skin rashes cleared up, as did her yeast overgrowth.

Many experts believe the body is healthiest when it is slightly alkaline rather than acidic. Mix the greens powder with water, hold your nose if you need to, and drink. Greens drinks we prefer are in Appendix B.

It Went In, But Did It Do Any Good?

The better your digestion, the easier it is to be at your ideal size. Unfortunately, good digestion isn't always a sure thing. Digestion becomes impaired by stress, and our digestive efficiency declines with age. It can also be harmed by other health and lifestyle factors. You don't want to miss one single nutrient from the food you eat.

Plus, proper and complete digestion can also reduce food and sugar cravings. So what can you do?

If you feel that your digestion is not ideal, digestive enzyme supplements may help. Many brands and formulations of digestive enzymes are available, and you want to take one that assists with protein, fat, and carbohydrate digestion. Only take digestive enzymes with meals. Experiment with different brands and formulations until you find one that works for you. Appendix B lists some choices for digestive enzymes.

If your intestinal flora is weak, you won't be able to assimilate nutrients well. Your "gut" needs a healthy stock of active bacteria. Without it, you could have diarrhea, constipation, or yeast overgrowth syndrome. Supplement with acidophilus-type supplements that contain active cultures.

Other Supplements Might Help

At one time or another it seems that every dietary supplement is claimed to assure weight loss. Here's a list of some that could help. But they aren't miraculous; they might simply aid your body in getting the nutrients it needs to lose weight.

- ◆ Conjugated linoleic acid, or CLA. This is a fatty acid that occurs naturally in meat, whole milk, and full-fat dairy products. This acid has been shown to promote the body's use of stored fat for energy and reduces the body's ability to store fat. It can be purchased as gel capsules. But if you eat meat and/or full-fat dairy products, you probably already consume adequate amounts.

- ◆ Free-form amino acids. If you eat complete high-quality protein at each meal, you already consume adequate amino acids. But if you eat as a vegetarian, an amino acid formula could be great for your health.

- ◆ Kelp, dulce, or bladderwrack are high in iodine, so if you're deficient in iodine, these could assist your thyroid in functioning better. But note: few people today are deficient in iodine, as it's added to salt and found in sea salt.

- ◆ Green tea contains caffeine and antioxidant catechins that promote thermogenesis. Drink three cups a day. It can be helpful if included in a healthy weight-loss program.

Eating natural unprocessed foods and taking healthful dietary supplements contribute to your overall health and may support your body in releasing fat. But it's unrealistic to hope that any single supplement can undo the overeating you've done for years.

Weight-Loss Supplements

So many advertisements promise instant weight loss. So many bottles of possibilities and promises line the shelves of health-food stores, grocery stores, and drugstores. The Internet and infomercials offer you endless opportunities to lose weight once and for all. The market is flooded with weight-loss supplements. But are any of them worth your time, hope, and money?

Some are; some aren't. So here's what you need to know about how the products work so you can make an informed decision.

Shakes. Diet shakes come in a can as a liquid or as a powder for you to mix with water or milk. The shakes are intended as meal replacements. They contain soy or whey protein and sugar or sweeteners with artificial flavorings for taste. Some contain added vitamins and minerals. You won't lose weight simply by drinking them. But you could consume fewer calories. Research shows, however, that drinking one's food can fool the body into consuming more calories than if a person ate a regular meal. Chewing food is a better weight-loss strategy. Soy is also indicated as suppressing thyroid production, which can slow your metabolism.

Bitter orange. Also known as citrus aurantium, bitter orange has replaced ephedra in some weight-loss supplements since the Food and Drug Administration (FDA) banned ephedra. It appears to be safer with fewer dramatic side effects than ephedra. Bitter orange stimulates the adrenal glands to rev up a person's metabolic rate and burn off body fat. Recently the FDA has placed bitter orange on its watch list because users are reporting undesirable side effects, such as increased blood pressure and heart palpitations.

CortiSlim. This is a brand-name product designed to reduce stress-induced cortisol levels while helping a person lose weight through a combination of bitter orange and caffeine. In effect, the product relaxes the body while hyping it up. You can find cortisol-lowering products that don't include bitter orange. Learn more about these in Chapter 8.

Bedtime potions. The labels claim you can shed extra pounds while you sleep. You're supposed to avoid eating anything for three hours before bed and take a spoonful or two of the potion right before you go to sleep. If these work at all, most likely it's because you won't be eating after dinner. Instead of purchasing the potion, don't eat three hours before bedtime. Product brand names include Calorad and Body Solutions.

Forslean. An award-winning extract of the coleus forskolii plant—an ayurvedic medicine herb. Forslean normalizes thyroid function, which helps you lose weight. The thyroid is the endocrine gland that regulates metabolism. Research indicates that forslean helps reduce blood pressure, reduces eczema and psoriasis, and reduces allergic reactions and asthma. Research from double-blind studies indicates the product is safe and effective for weight loss. The best delivery system for forslean is a transdermal patch. Forslean is not a magic bullet, so you'll still need to eat balanced meals, eat 0–5, and get regular exercise along with wearing the patch. See Appendix B on where to purchase.

If you find other weight-loss supplements, be sure to do your research before you buy. You can expect the website to praise the product along with published testimonials, so dig deeper. Check out the Internet for any negative comments about the product. Check out the scientific research and any FDA comments or warnings. Then decide whether you want to give the product a try.

Balance, Balance, Balance

Yes, supplements can help you make sure that you're obtaining all the essential amino acids, necessary sugars, essential fatty acids, and micronutrients. But think of them as "supplements," not as substitutes for good food. They're not a short cut to weight loss. One seminar participant, Alice, admitted she was hoping there were pills she could take so that she could keep bingeing on the sugars and starches she loved. Too bad that won't work. She deserves praise for her honesty, but she won't be able to release her weight.

Eat a balanced diet as described in Chapter 12 and use the supplements for extra support, not the main course. Recommendations for supplements are in Appendix B.

The Least You Need to Know

♦ Taking dietary supplements can help to ensure that you receive adequate amounts of nutrients to support your weight loss.

♦ Nutritional supplements support your body in releasing fat, reduce cravings, and maintain energy levels.

♦ Some weight-loss supplements work well when combined with proper eating and regular exercise, but many are more hype than help.

♦ Beware, some weight-loss supplements are a waste of money and only marginally safe, if at all.

Part 4

Eating for Weight Loss

When it comes to the question of what's for dinner, make your selection from the menus in this part of the book. Four basic weight-loss programs have stood the test of time: low-glycemic, low-carb, low-calorie, and low-fat. Learn which one will work best for you, based on your health concerns, your dieting history, and your lifestyle. You'll find menu suggestions for two weeks of delicious and healthy eating for each of the weight-loss programs, but don't mix and match. Instead, choose a program and stick with it for three or four months and give your program time to work for you.

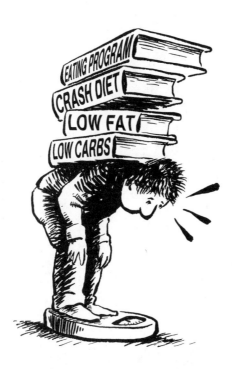

12

Designing Your Healthy Weight-Loss Plan

In This Chapter

♦ Designing an eating plan that works for you

♦ Eating the basics first

♦ Understanding the Food Pyramid for Weight Loss

♦ The challenge of vegetarianism

Now that you've gotten this far into the book, you're probably thinking, "So, when do we eat?" You've learned a wealth of detailed information about how your body works, nutrition, and the factors affecting weight. Now you want to put it all together into a weight-loss eating plan that works for you.

Your eating approach must be tailored to meet your needs, which is why you'll be able to assess which of four eating plans is right for you— low-glycemic, low-carb, low-calorie, or low-fat.

In this chapter, you learn what basic foods are included in all the plans based on the New Food Pyramid for Weight Loss and how to use the Plate Method for serving your food. So let's get started!

You Need to Like What You Eat

First and foremost, eat foods that are the most appealing to you. If you don't like the foods you eat, you won't be able to eat beautifully and sensuously. You still need to eat the nutrition basics—vegetables, fruit, animal protein, and fats. But you can select the types of meats, fruit, vegetables, and fats that give you the most pleasure, or the ones that are in season where you live, or even the ones that your family is more likely to enjoy. Within any of the four eating programs we offer, you have plenty of choices as to the specific foods to eat.

Lean Lingo

Only eat food that you enjoy. You do not need to eat unappealing foods to get to your ideal size, nor should you. Make your eating a pleasurable and sensuous delight.

So eat the specific foods that really appeal to you. No, we're not encouraging you to eat a quart of ice cream for dinner. But we do mean this: if you have never met a green pea that you like, don't eat green peas. Ditto for cauliflower or onions. Eat foods you do like that have comparable nutritional value.

How many oddball diets have you read about or maybe experimented with? Shellie, age 48, was a classic obsessive dieter. Over the years, she tried special diets that promoted the following:

◆ Rice cakes (She called them "cardboard sandwiches.")

◆ Grapefruit ("An orange with a sour disposition.")

◆ Yogurt ("Milk that's gone bad.")

◆ Watermelon ("Lots of water, lots of sugar, where's the food?")

◆ Cabbage soup ("Not bad for the first 20 bowls.")

It took considerable effort to persuade Shellie that she could lose weight and actually eat what she liked … including chocolate and treat foods. Shellie, now 20 pounds lighter, makes her dieting past sound funny, but her story is all too common.

In your efforts to get to your ideal size, no plan will work for a lifetime if you have to eat yucky foods. Shellie still eats cabbage soup, just not bowls and bowls of it. Too much of even a good thing is not a good thing.

Balance Is Everything

A friend born and raised in France but now living in the United States made this observation: "What amazes me about Americans is that they eat the same foods day after day. Why, in France, we wouldn't think of eating the same food twice in the same week." (As you probably know, the French don't have anywhere near the overweight and obesity issues plaguing the U.S. population.) We like her philosophy of eating a wide variety of foods. This reduces boredom of the palate and also gives you many more types of nutrients from your foods.

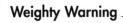

Weighty Warning

Research shows that eating the same types of food day after day can bring on food allergies or sensitivities—one more good reason to eat a wide variety of foods.

The New Food Pyramid for Weight Loss

Two health care practitioners at the University of Utah Diabetes Center, Dana Clarke, M.D., C.D.E., and Joan Clark, M.S., R.D., C.D.E., and one of the co-authors of this book, have developed a new food pyramid that's based on their research with patients. It's called the Food Guide Pyramid for Type 2 Diabetes & Weight Management.

It isn't surprising that the new Food Guide Pyramid was developed both for persons with diabetes and for people who want to lose weight. Both groups of people need to keep their blood sugar levels in the safe range. For people who want to lose weight, this helps prevent the body from storing fat and reduces the likelihood of insulin resistance, which also causes weight gain.

The pyramid helps you to understand the basics of healthy eating, and the underlying structure works for all four of the eating programs described in the following four chapters. Here's the info on the food pyramid from top to bottom.

Weighty Warning

When referring to the Food Guide Pyramid, remember to be careful about your serving sizes. Too much food is still too much food, no matter which eating plan you prefer. A great rule of thumb is to never, never, never overeat. As you read earlier in this book, overeating leads to insulin resistance. Stay true to your body—eat 0–5.

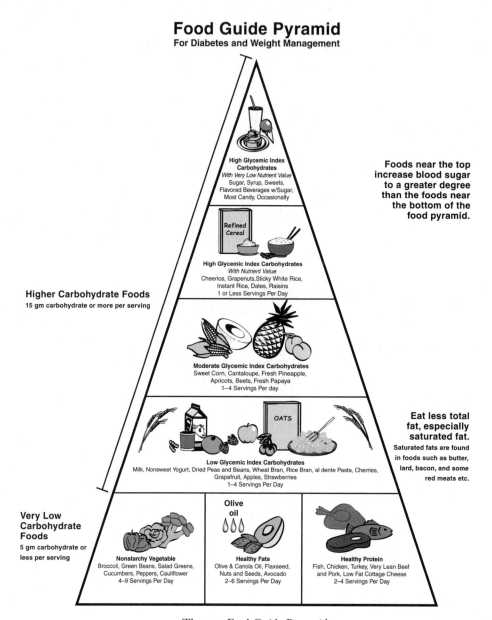

The new Food Guide Pyramid.

◆ At the top of the Food Guide Pyramid are the foods to eat sparingly and infrequently. These are high-glycemic carbohydrates that have little to no nutritional value, such as syrup, sweets, and baked goods that have a glycemic index value of 72 or above.

◆ The next level down includes high-glycemic carbohydrates that have some nutritional value. The list includes breakfast cereals and sticky white rice. You can eat up to 2 servings a day. A serving size is ½ cup.

◆ Next are medium-glycemic carbohydrates such as apricots, papayas, fresh pineapple, and raisins. You can eat 2–4 servings a day. A serving size is ½ cup.

◆ From here on down through the pyramid are the foods you want to eat for best weight-loss results. At the fourth level are the low-glycemic carbohydrates. They include dairy products, such as milk, non-sweetened yogurt, legumes, 100 percent whole-grain kernels, rice bran, yams, sweet potatoes, and pasta cooked al dente. This level also includes lower-glycemic fruits, such as pears, apples, dates, oranges, cherries, and all others that are low-glycemic. A serving size is ½ cup. You can eat 2–4 servings per day of foods from level four.

◆ At the bottom of the Food Guide Pyramid, at level 5, are low-carbohydrate foods. These include all non-starchy vegetables, such as broccoli, spinach, green beans, carrots, and asparagus. Eat 4–9 servings a day. A serving size is ½ cup cooked or 1 cup raw.

◆ Next to the vegetables are the healthy fats, such as avocados, olive oil, and nuts and seeds. Eat 2–6 servings a day. Serving size varies here. For an avocado, use ¼ small avocado; for nuts and seeds, 6 nuts or 2 tablespoons of nuts and seeds; for oils and fats, one serving is one teaspoon.

◆ The last item on the bottom level is healthy protein, including lean meats, seafood, poultry, and low-fat cottage cheese. Have 2–4 servings per day. A serving size is 3–4 ounces or ¼ cup cottage cheese.

So, to lose weight, eat mostly from the two lowest levels of the Food Guide Pyramid. Eat infrequently from the upper three levels.

We love this food guide. It makes losing weight easy. You can't go wrong eating foods in moderate serving sizes from the bottom two levels. Try taking the Food Guide Pyramid with you to the grocery store. Purchase foods in the bottom three levels, with an emphasis on the bottom two.

Body of Knowledge

Where do eggs fit in? They're at the bottom of the Food Guide Pyramid in healthy protein. A serving is two eggs, or one egg and 2 egg whites, or can be 3–4 egg whites, based on whether or not you're eating on the low-fat program.

Perhaps you're wondering whether eating foods from the bottom two levels of the Food Guide Pyramid can satisfy your appetite. These foods generally stay in your stomach longer, are generally more bulky, and help to keep your blood sugar more stable. Eating this way helps with satiety. We think you'll love the results—your clothes will be fitting better.

Also remember that you don't need to totally give up your treat foods, but to eat them sparingly. In the beginning of your weight-loss program, however, you might want to avoid the goodies if they have been "trigger" foods for you in the past. Trigger foods tend to be psychologically addictive. You know, the foods that can cause you to keep going back for more and more and more. After eating more foods at the bottom of the food pyramid, many people find they crave salads and vegetables more than they desire the high-glycemic and fattening goodies.

Sizing Up Your Plate

If you're a visual person and have been known to eat based on what your eyes can take in rather than on what your stomach can accommodate, the Plate Method could be just what you need.

The Plate Method is designed to show you what and about how much you need to eat to lose weight. So here's what to put on your plate (see the figure that follows):

◆ Fill just about half of your plate with nonstarchy vegetables. These include all nonstarchy vegetables located on the bottom of the pyramid.

◆ Fill about one quarter of your plate with low-glycemic starches, fruit, or dairy products.

Body of Knowledge

By filling almost half your plate with vegetables and having another quarter for fruit, you'll be sure to eat the recommended amount of 5–10 servings of vegetables and fruit every day.

◆ A little less than ¼ (20–25%) of your plate is for lean protein, including meats, seafood, or poultry. Figure that ¼ is about 3 to 4 ounces.

◆ The remaining wedge of your plate, or about 5% or less, is for healthy fats, such as olive oil, avocados, and nuts and seeds.

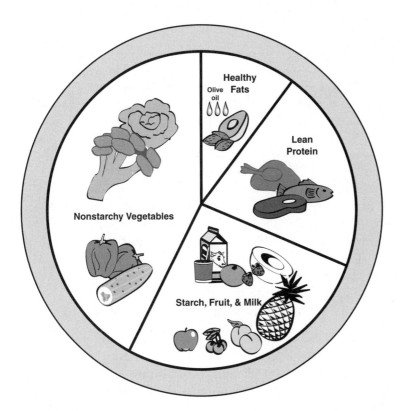

The Plate Method.

In actuality, your plate won't look exactly like this. Usually, the fats will be part of your foods, as dressing for your vegetables, or as nuts and seeds sprinkled over your salad. And, as you know, oils run and spread all over the other foods.

The Plate Method works for all the eating programs and also is great for weight-loss maintenance. You'll be keeping your portion sizes moderate, and you'll be eating healthfully. Teach your children to use the Plate Method. Most likely, they'll relate better to the plate than the food pyramid. You can even have them make meal suggestions based on the Plate Method!

Try it a few times. Serve food onto your plate with a sense of how it should look according to the preceding formula. In no time at all, you will be using it—even at challenging eating situations, such as buffets, potluck dinners, Grandma's house, or with your children.

Weighty Warning _____

Compare the size of a modern dinner plate to one in Grandma's china set. A modern dinner plate has 36 square inches of surface area, compared to 33 on Grandma's. Simply by using a smaller-sized plate, you'll eat less food at every meal. Eating all the food on those extra 3 square inches three times a day can add up quickly to increase your waistline by 3 more inches.

And one final Plate Method suggestion … serve dinner from the stove, not family-style with bowls of food at the table. This discourages overeating and encourages controlled eating based on feelings of real hunger and satisfaction. This might clash with family tradition, but try it and see whether it doesn't help limit unconsciously eating second and third helpings.

The Trials of a Strict Vegetarian Diet

If you're a vegetarian, you've noticed that the New Food Guide Pyramid doesn't fit well for you. If you have chosen to be a vegetarian but eat cheese, dairy, eggs, and fish, you can use the menus in the following chapters by substituting one of these for the meat suggestions. Cheese, eggs, and fish are high-quality proteins that can be prepared in innumerable ways. Just make sure that you emphasize vegetables and fruits. If you are a total vegetarian or vegan, however, meaning you eat no animal products, your protein choices are far more limited. Getting enough high-quality protein is challenging, if not impossible.

Weighty Warning _____

Recent studies suggest that women who eat low-quality protein, such as beans and rice, do not lose weight because the thyroid reacts as though the body is starving. Recent studies also report some concern about possible health risks associated with eating high amounts of processed soy, such as thyroid and hormonal imbalances. So be careful with your soy powders and with protein bars that are high in soy protein isolate. Experts recommend that you eat them only once or twice a week.

Many vegetarians consume soy products as their primary source of protein. Soy isn't a complete protein because it doesn't have adequate amounts of methionine, one of the essential amino acids. To obtain complete protein, soy products need to be eaten with grains through food combining. Even with food combining, consuming 20 to 25 percent protein, 20-30% fat, and only 45-50 percent carbs will be a challenge.

The Right Eating Program for You

In the following four chapters are four different eating plans. As you read through the plans, notice that the menus for each plan are based on the same foods, but we've varied the amounts of some foods to satisfy the needs of the eating plans. For example, a person on a low-fat plan would eat leaner meats and use less butter than on other plans.

Here are some guidelines for deciding which one will work best for you:

Low-glycemic Eating Program

Choose this program if …

- ◆ You have elevated blood sugar levels.

- ◆ You have hypoglycemia.

- ◆ You're allergic or food-sensitive to wheat or gluten.

- ◆ You have metabolic syndrome, also known as Syndrome X, with elevated blood sugar levels, high triglyceride levels, high blood pressure, and weight gain around the waist and abdomen.

- ◆ You've tried all the other diet plans, and nothing's worked for you.

Low-Carb Eating Program

Choose this program if …

- ◆ You've tried low-fat diets, and they haven't worked for you.

- ◆ You've tried low-calorie diets, and they haven't worked for you.

- ◆ You don't have diabetes, metabolic syndrome, or hypoglycemia.

Weighty Warning

If you simply love to overeat, none of these programs will work well for you. So choose the plan that appeals to you the most and be careful to eat 0-5. Remember that eating 0-5 is a status symbol all by itself. So is the body size you'll attain.

Low-Calorie Eating Program

Choose this program if …

◆ You are comfortable with counting your calories and keeping track of them throughout the day.

◆ You have no significant health issues, such as metabolic syndrome, high blood pressure, high triglycerides, elevated blood sugar levels, high cholesterol, diabetes, or heart disease.

Low-Fat Eating Program

Choose this program if …

◆ You're already accustomed to eating low-fat.

◆ Your doctor or healthcare practitioner has recommended that you eat a low-fat diet.

◆ You have cardiac problems or high cholesterol.

◆ You want to lower your triglyceride levels.

After you've made your eating program selection, stick with it for a month or two so you can clearly know whether it works for you or not. If it doesn't, then you can switch to a different plan. But before you do, make sure that you are following the recommendations in this book for eating 0–5 and boosting your metabolism.

The Least You Need to Know

◆ Eat balanced meals consisting of foods that you enjoy.

◆ Use the New Food Guide Pyramid to make food selections.

◆ The menu plans for the four weight-loss programs are based on the Food Guide Pyramid in this chapter.

◆ Use the Plate Method for serving your food at mealtimes and for teaching your children how to eat.

Chapter 3

The Low-Glycemic Eating Plan

In This Chapter

◆ Eating based on the glycemic index

◆ Managing your blood sugar levels

◆ Working with your hormones to release fat

Eating based on the glycemic index works. It's the newest kid on the weight-loss block, and the most scientifically up-to-date. That's why we put this eating program first.

Using the glycemic index and glycemic load as a basis for weight loss can be complex. But by following the daily menus in this chapter, you'll find it easy. Soon, you'll become a pro at planning your meals and snacks.

Benefits of Low-Glycemic Eating

Eating low-glycemic is excellent for you if:

- You've failed with other eating plans, including low-calorie, low-fat, and low-carb.

- You have diabetes or hypoglycemia.

- You have metabolic syndrome, meaning that you have the following: elevated tri-glycerides, elevated blood sugar levels, and weight gain around your mid-section.

- You have high stress levels.

- You carry extra weight around your waist and abdomen.

- You have high blood pressure or heart disease.

- You have a weakened immune system.

- You have an autoimmune condition such as arthritis, MS, fibromyalgia, or chronic fatigue syndrome.

- You are metabolically resistant to weight loss.

- You've yo-yo dieted for years.

- You want to retain lean muscle and lose body fat.

Thinspiration

Eating low-glycemic is great for your health. Many people who don't need to lose weight eat low-glycemic to support their health. After you've reached your ideal size, you can continue to eat low-glycemic to maintain your weight but increase your daily glycemic load.

As you can see from reading the preceding list, eating low-glycemic can help to improve many health conditions. It's also great if your metabolism is slow or sluggish.

The Hormone Factor

One fabulous benefit of eating low-glycemic is that you can keep your body's level of the hormone insulin at a healthy level. When your insulin level is too high, usually after eating fluffy white starches or a heavy dose of sugar, the body produces more insulin than usual and causes your body to store fat. Not exactly what you want when you're trying to lose weight. In fact, it's not what you want when you aren't trying to lose weight.

Another hormone that plays a big role in weight gain is the stress hormone cortisol. When it's high, your levels of insulin are also elevated, and the opposite is also true. So you'll lose weight more easily when your stress is low. Eating low-glycemic foods can help keep insulin and cortisol levels lower. Eating high-glycemic foods can increase cortisol/stress levels.

The low-glycemic eating program works with your biology, your hormones, and your health to help you release body fat more easily.

The Glycemic Load

The glycemic load tells you how many of the carbs you're eating are factored in with the glycemic index. The formula is as follows:

> Serving of carbs in grams × glycemic index ÷ 100. Your total for each day needs to be between 50 and 75. In the menus that follow, we give you the glycemic index and glycemic load for each serving of carbohydrates, so you can use these values when you eat out or in other eating situations.

Week 1 Menus for Low-Glycemic Eating Plan

As you read through the menus below, you'll notice that some of the foods don't have GI and GL listings. That's because those foods don't contain a significant amount of carbohydrates to be listed in the glycemic index.

Monday:

Breakfast:
Broiled Canadian Bacon (2 ounces) with Tomato Parmesan (1 med. Tomato sliced, and 2 tsp. Parmesan) GI = 38, GL = 4
Corn Tortilla (1 small) GI = 68, GL =10
Fresh Peach Slices (1 peach) GI = 28, GL = 4 with
Yogurt, plain/low-fat (6 ounces) GI = 36, GL = 3

Breakfast Glycemic Load: 21

Snack:
Fresh Baby Carrots and Sugar Snap Peas (1 cup) GI = 16, GL = 1
Toasted Peanuts (2 TB.)

Snack Glycemic Load: 1

Lunch:
Spinach-Celery (2 cups chopped) with Whole-Grain Pasta (⅓ cup cooked) Salad GI = 32, GL = 10
Red Grapes (⅓ cup) GI = 46, GL = 7
Grilled Salmon (3 oz.)
Vinaigrette Dressing (2 TB.)

Lunch Glycemic Load: 17

Snack:
Fresh Pineapple Chunks (⅔ cup) GI = 66, GL = 10
Dates (2) GI = 50, GL = 6

Snack Glycemic Load: 16

Dinner:
Lemon-Pepper Chicken Breast (3 oz.)
Steamed Broccoli Spears (2 cups) GI = 10, GL = 1
Feta Cheese (1 TB.)
Baked Yam (¾ cup) GI = 37, GL = 13
Butter (1 tsp.)

Dinner Glycemic Load: 14

Snack:
Fresh Cantaloupe Slices (1 cup) GI = 65, GL = 8

Snack Glycemic Load: 8

Total Glycemic Load for Monday: 77

Tuesday:

Breakfast:
Whole-wheat Pita (1 oz.) GI = 57, GL = 10 with Chicken (2 oz.)
Tomato, Onion, and Pepper (1 cup) GI = 10, GL = 1 and Cheese (1 oz.)
Cucumber Spears (1 cup)
Fresh Whole Strawberries (1 cup) GI = 40, GL = 6
Unsweetened Whipped Cream (1 tsp.)

Breakfast Glycemic Load: 17

Snack:
Avocado (⅛ large)
Celery (1 cup) GI = 0, GL = 0

Snack Glycemic Load: 0

Lunch:
Grilled Pork Tenderloin (3 oz.)
Fresh Steamed Green Beans (1 cup) and Almond Slices (1 TB.)
Spinach/Romaine Greens (1 cup) and Vinaigrette Dressing (2 TB.)
Baked Winter Squash (¾ cup) GI = 37, GL = 4 with Apple Slices and Cinnamon
 (¼ cup) GI = 38, GL = 3

Lunch Glycemic Load: 7

Snack:
Pure Ice Cream (¼ cup) GI = 38, GL = 3
Almonds (6)

Snack Glycemic Load: 3

Dinner:
Beef Tenderloin (3 oz.) with Sun-dried Tomatoes (2 TB.)
Asparagus Spears (1 cup)
Wild Rice and Herbs (½ cup) GI = 58, GL = 11
Mint Iced Tea with Lime

Dinner Glycemic Load: 11

Snack:
Cantaloupe (1 cup) GI = 65, GL = 10
Chamomile Tea (iced or hot plain or with Stevia with FOS)

Snack Glycemic Load: 10

Total Glycemic Load for Tuesday: 48

Wednesday:

Breakfast:
Cheese (1 oz.) Pepper and Herb Omelet (1 egg, 2 egg whites)
Whole-wheat Tortilla (6-in.) GI = 30, GL = 8
Salsa GI = 36, GL = 1
Honeydew Melon Chunks (1 cup) GI = 65, GL = 4

Breakfast Glycemic Load: 13

Snack:
Crispy Broccoli and Cauliflower Flowerets (1 cup)
Salad Dressing (1 TB.)

Snack Glycemic Load: 0

Lunch:
Hearty Beef Vegetable Soup with
  Beef (2 oz.)
  Tomatoes, Carrots, Onions (1 cup) GI = 42, GL = 4
  Navy or Pinto Beans (⅓ cup) GI = 38, GL – 5
  Pearled Barley (⅓ cup) GI = 42, GL = 6
Fresh Mango Slices (½ cup) with Whipped Cream (1 tsp.) GI = 51, GL = 8

Lunch Glycemic Load: 23

Snack:
Dark Chocolate (1 oz. square) GI = 48, GL = 8
Green Tea (decaf, iced, or hot)

Snack Glycemic Load: 8

Dinner:
Barbequed Turkey (3 oz.)
Corn on the Cob (5-in.) GI = 60, GL = 9
Summer Squash (1 cup) and Feta (1 tsp.)
Vinaigrette Coleslaw (1 cup) with Cranberries (2 TB. dried) GI = 52, GL = 6
Lemonade (sugar-free sweetened with Stevia with FOS)

Dinner Glycemic Load: 15

Snack:
Fresh Apple Slices (1 small apple) GI = 38, GL = 6 with Peanut Butter (½ TB.)

Snack Glycemic Load: 6

Total Glycemic Load for Wednesday: 65

Thursday:

Breakfast:
Grilled Sirloin Strips (2 oz.)
Zucchini, Tomato, Onion (2 cups) GI = 18, GL = 2 and Parmesan (2 TB.)
Hearty Whole-grain Bread (1 slice) GI = 52, GL = 8
Apricots (3 fresh) GI = 57, GL = 7

Breakfast Glycemic Load: 17

Snack:
Cucumber Wedges (1 cup) and Feta Cheese (1 TB.)

Snack Glycemic Load: 0

Lunch:
Tuna Lettuce Wraps (3 oz. tuna, 1 tsp. mayonnaise, ½ tsp. mustard, and 4 large
  Romaine leaves)
Spiced Whole Baby Beets (½ cup, no sugar added) GI = 64, GL = 5
Long-grain Brown Rice (⅓ cup) GI = 61, GL = 9 with Sunflower Seeds (1 tsp.)
Fresh/Frozen Bing Cherries (¼ cup) GI = 22, GL = 2 and Plain Non-fat Yogurt (6 oz.)
  GI = 14, GL = 2

Lunch Glycemic Load: 18

Snack:
Pure Ice Cream (⅓ cup) GI = 31, GL = 3
Freshly brewed Decaf (no added sugar)

Snack Glycemic Load: 3

Dinner:
Whole-grain Chicken Fajita (2 oz. diced cooked chicken, 1 oz. cheese, peppers, ½ cup
  cooked onions and one 6-in. whole-grain flour tortilla) GI = 30, GL = 8
Salsa (¼ cup) GI = 36, GL = 1
Celery, Carrot (1½ cups), and Olive (6 olives) Relish Tray GI = 23, GL = 2

Dinner Glycemic Load: 11

Snack:
Fresh Apple Slices (1 small apple) GI = 36 , GL = 6
Walnuts (4)

Snack Glycemic Load: 6

Total Glycemic Load for Thursday: 55

Friday:

Breakfast:
Whole-wheat Pita with Cheese and Nuts
  Pita (1 oz. or ½ small) GI = 57, GL = 10
  Feta Cheese (1 oz.)
  Cottage Cheese (2 TB.)
  Almonds (4, chopped)
Fresh Whole Strawberries (2 cups) GI = 40, GL = 10

Breakfast Glycemic Load: 20

Snack:
Grape Tomatoes (1 cup) GI = 32, GL = 2

Snack Glycemic Load: 2

Lunch:
Grilled Chicken (3 oz.)
Roasted Corn on the Cob (1–5-in.) GI = 60, GL = 9
Fresh Seasoned Green Beans (1 cup)
Spinach-Orange Salad (1 cup spinach and ¼ cup orange slices) GI = 42, GL = 2
Vinaigrette Dressing (1 TB.)

Lunch Glycemic Load: 11

Snack:
Fresh Watermelon (1½ cups) GI = 72, GL = 4
Herbal Tea

Snack Glycemic Load: 4

Dinner:
Seafood Kabobs
  Large Shrimp (4), Scallops (4)
  Pea Pods and Onion, and Red Bell Peppers (½ cup)
  Pineapple Chunks (¼ cup) GI = 66, GL = 5
  Soy Sauce, Spices
Julienne Carrots (¼ cup) GI = 49, GL = 2 and Black Rice (⅓ cup) GI = 58, GL = 9

Dinner Glycemic Load: 14

Snack:
Pure Ice Cream (⅓ cup) GI = 31, GL = 3
Herbal Tea

Snack Glycemic Load: 3

Total Glycemic Load for Friday: 54

Saturday:

Breakfast:
Steel-cut Oats (1 cup cooked oats) GI = 47, GL = 14 with Peaches and Cinnamon
  (⅓ cup peaches) GI = 42, GL = 4
Cottage Cheese (¾ cup)
Raw Almonds (6)

Breakfast Glycemic Load: 18

Snack:
Sugar Snap Peas (1 cup) and Carrot Strips (½ cup) GI = 47, GL = 2

Snack Glycemic Load: 2

Lunch:
Spinach–Whole-grain Pasta Salad with Chicken and Garbanzo Beans
  Spinach (2 cups)   Pasta (⅓ cup cooked al dente) GI = 32, GL = 5
  Chicken (3 oz.)   Garbanzo Beans (⅓ cup) GI = 31, GL = 5
  Ranch Salad Dressing (1 TB.)   Red Wine Vinegar (unlimited)

Lunch Glycemic Load: 10

Snack:
Dark Chocolate (1 oz.) GI = 48, GL = 8   Fresh Apple (½) GI = 36, GL = 3
Herbal Tea

Snack Glycemic Load: 11

Dinner:
Grilled Tenderloin and Vegetable Kabobs
  Onions (½ cup)   Whole Mushrooms (½ cup)
  Tomato Wedges (½ cup)   Tenderloin Steak, cubed (3 oz.)
Black Beans with Green Onions (½ cup) GI = 30, GL = 5
Berry Parfait
  Blueberries (⅓ cup) GI = 40, GL = 3
  Raspberries (⅓ cup) GI = 38, GL = 2
  Whipped Cream (1 TB.)

Dinner Glycemic Load: 10

Snack:
Fresh Bartlett Pear GI = 38, GL = 4   Herbal Tea

Snack Glycemic Load: 4

Total Glycemic Load for Saturday: 55

Sunday:

Breakfast:
Vegetable/Cheese Egg Omelet
  Raw Veggies, diced (1 cup)   Grated Cheese (½ oz.)
  Egg (1) and Egg Whites (2)
Hearty Whole-grain Toast (1 slice) GI = 52, GL = 8
Fresh Grapefruit (1 small whole) GI = 25, GL = 3
Butter (1 tsp.)

Breakfast Glycemic Load: 11

Snack:
Edamame (green soybeans, lightly cooked, ½ cup) and Filberts (10)
Herbal Tea

Snack Glycemic Load: 0

Lunch:
Baked Cod   Steamed Asparagus Tips (½ cup)
Tomato/Onion Vinaigrette Salad (1 cup) GI = 32, GL = 2
New Red Potatoes with Skin (5 oz.) GI = 78, GL = 16

Lunch Glycemic Load: 18

Snack:
Dates (3) GI = 50, GL = 4   Herbal Tea

Snack Glycemic Load: 4

Dinner:
Taco Salad
  Cheese, shredded, (1 oz.)   Seasoned Turkey Strips (2 oz.)
  Avocado (⅛ chopped)
  Onion, Tomatoes, Peppers, Dark Greens (3 cups) GI = 10, GL = 1
  Salsa (¼ cup) GI = 36, GL = 1
Whole-grain Pita Bread (½ small, cut into triangles and baked until crispy) GI = 57,
  GL = 10

Dinner Glycemic Load: 12

Snack:
Dried Apricots (8 halves) GI = 30, GL = 4   Almonds (8 raw)

Snack Glycemic Load: 4

Total Glycemic Load for Sunday: 49

Week 2 Menus for Low-Glycemic Eating Plan

Monday:

Breakfast:
Museli or All-Bran Cereal (½ cup) GI = 30, GL = 4
Milk, 1 percent (6 oz.) GI = 32, GL = 3
Banana Slices (1 medium) GI = 52, GL = 12
Boiled Egg (1)
Breakfast Glycemic Load: 19

Snack:
Grape Tomatoes (1 cup) GI = 10, GL = 1
Snack Glycemic Load: 1

Lunch:
Shrimp, Lima Bean, and Apple-Nut Salad
  Shrimp (3 oz.)   Romaine Lettuce, Onion, Celery (3 cups)
  Lima Beans (½ cup) GI = 31, GL = 5   Raw Cashews (6)
  Feta Cheese (½ oz.)   Vinaigrette Salad Dressing (2 TB.)
  Apple Slices (1 medium apple) GI = 38, GL = 7
Lunch Glycemic Load: 12

Snack:
Dark Chocolate (1 oz.) GI = 48, GL = 8   Herbal Tea
Snack Glycemic Load: 8

Dinner:
Apricot-Chicken Stir Fry
  Chicken (3 oz.), Dried Apricot Halves (6), diced GI = 30, GL = 4
  Onion Slices and Red and Green Pepper Slices (2 cups)
  Brown Rice (⅓ cup) GI = 61, GL = 22
Dinner Glycemic Load: 26

Snack:
Peach Yogurt Parfait
  Sliced Peaches (1 fresh) GI = 42, GL = 5
  Plain Non-fat Yogurt (½ cup) GI = 32, GL = 2
Snack Glycemic Load: 7

Total Glycemic Load for Monday: 73

Tuesday:

Breakfast:
Broiled Ham and Tomato with Cheddar
  Ham (2 oz.), Cheddar Cheese Shredded (1 oz.) on
  Tomato Slices, Broiled (1 medium tomato) GI = 10, GL = 1
Black Beans with Fresh Tarragon (½ cup) GI = 30, GL = 5
Honeydew Melon Slices (1½ cups) GI = 65, GL = 14

Breakfast Glycemic Load: 20

Snack:
Sugar Snap Peas and Celery   Cashew Nuts (6)

Snack Glycemic Load: 0

Lunch:
Turkey, Pecan, and Pear on Baby Greens
  Turkey (cut into strips, 3 oz.), Pecan Halves (4), Fresh Pear (sliced, 1 medium)
    GI = 38, GL = 7
  Baby Greens (2 cups)
Coarsely Ground Whole-grain Toast (1 slice) GI = 61, GL = 9
Vinaigrette Salad Dressing (2 TB.)

Lunch Glycemic Load: 16

Snack:
Red Grapes (17 small) GI = 43, GL = 17   Herbal Tea

Snack Glycemic Load: 17

Dinner:
Spaghetti Squash with Sauce
  Squash (2 cups)
  Spaghetti Sauce (½ cup) GI = 25, GL = 2
  Parmesan Cheese (1 oz.)
  Lean Ground Meat (2 oz.)
Fresh Blueberries (¾ cup) GI = 57, GL = 10 with Whipped Cream (1 TB.)

Dinner Glycemic Load: 12

Snack:
Pure Ice Cream (⅓ cup) GI = 32, GL = 3   Herbal Tea

Snack Glycemic Load: 3

Total Glycemic Load for Tuesday: 68

Wednesday:

Breakfast:

Rolled Barley and Bran with Dried Apricots and Nuts

 Rolled Barley or Thick-cut Oats (¼ cup dry/½ cup cooked) GI = 48, GL = 7

 Unprocessed Wheat Bran (¼ cup dry/½ cup cooked) GI = 25, GL = 4

 Dried Apricots (8 halves, diced) GI = 30, GL = 4

 Almonds (12)

Protein Fruit Shake

 Whey Protein Powder (2 TB.) (with no carbohydrates)

 Banana Slices (½ cup) GI = 52, GL = 4   Strawberries (½ cup) GI = 57, GL = 5

 Water and Ice (1 cup)   If desired, Stevia to sweeten

Breakfast Glycemic Load: 24

Snack:

Carrot Sticks, raw (1 cup) GI = 47, GL = 4

Snack Glycemic Load: 4

Lunch:

Roasted Chicken and Vegetables

 Chicken (3 oz.)

 Carrots, Fresh Green Beans, and Tomato (1 cup cooked) GI = 22, GL = 1

Pea and Whole Pasta Salad

 Chopped Fresh Spinach and Onion (1 cup)   Peas (¼ cup) GI = 48, GL = 2

 Pasta, cooked al dente (⅓ cup) GI = 52, GL = 8   Herbs and Spices

 Vinaigrette Dressing (2 TB.)

Lunch Glycemic Load: 11

Snack:

Dark Chocolate (1 oz. square) GI = 48, GL = 8   Herbal Tea

Snack Glycemic Load: 8

Dinner:

Haddock Fillet with Herbs (3 oz.)   Vinaigrette Coleslaw (1 cup) GI = 10, GL = 1

Summer Squash (1 cup, cooked) GI = 10, GL = 1

Spicy Sweet Potato Wedges (½ cup) GI = 61, GL = 9

Dinner Glycemic Load: 11

Snack:

Hot Cocoa (1 cup sweetened with Stevia)   1 percent or Skim Milk (1 cup) GI = 32, GL = 4

 Unsweetened Cocoa Powder (1 tsp.)

Snack Glycemic Load: 4

Total Glycemic Load for Wednesday: 62

Thursday:

Breakfast:

Vegetable Egg Scramble with Cheese and Bacon Bits

  Egg (1) and Egg Whites (2)

  Onions, Tomatoes, Spinach, chopped and mixed with eggs (1 cup) GI = 10, GL = 1

  Cheese, shredded on top egg dish (½ oz.)

  Crispy bacon, drained well, crumbled on egg dish (1 slice)

Strawberries and Yogurt

  Strawberries (2 cups) GI = 40, GL = 10

  Yogurt, Non-fat Plain (1 cup) GI = 32, GL = 4

Breakfast Glycemic Load: 15

Snack:

Broccoli and Cauliflower Flowerets (1 cup)   Ranch Dressing (1 TB.)

Snack Glycemic Load: 0

Lunch:

Red Beans, Spinach, and Long Grain Brown Rice with Turkey

  Spinach and Onions, chopped (2 cups)   Red Beans (½ cup) GI = 45, GL = 10

  Brown Rice (⅓ cup) GI = 50, GL = 7   Turkey, cut lengthwise (2 oz.)

  Feta Cheese, sprinkled on top (1 TB.)

Iced Tea

Lunch Glycemic Load: 17

Snack:

Apple Slices (1 medium apple) GI = 38, GL = 6   Filberts (10)

Snack Glycemic Load: 6

Dinner:

Grilled Chicken Breast with Sun-dried Tomatoes

  Chicken (3 oz.)   Sun-dried Tomatoes (2 TB.) GI = 36, GL = 3

Whole-grain Penne Rigate pasta, cooked al dente (½ cup) GI = 44, GI = 9

Pasta Sauce (¼ cup) GI = 36, GL = 1

Sugar Snap Pea, Celery, and Sweet Red Pepper Salad (2 cups)

Green Olives (5)

Vinaigrette Dressing (2 TB.)

Dinner Glycemic Load: 13

Snack:

Dark Chocolate (1 oz. square) GI = 48, GL = 8   Herbal Tea

Snack Glycemic Load: 8

Total Glycemic Load for Thursday: 59

Friday:

Breakfast:

Vegetable Egg Scramble and Corn Tortilla
  Egg (1) and Egg Whites (2)
  Chopped Tomatoes, Onions, Spinach (1 cup) GI = 10, GL = 1
  Small Corn Tortilla (1) GI = 65, GL = 8
  Salsa (2–4 TB.) GI = 10, GL = 1
Red Beans and Spices (½ cup) GI = 45, GL = 10
Kiwi Slices (½ cup) GI = 38, GL = 5

Breakfast Glycemic Load: 25

Snack:

Watermelon, cubed (1 cup) GI = 72, GL = 7   Iced or Hot Herbal Tea

Snack Glycemic Load: 7

Lunch:

Shrimp and Snow Pea, Spinach Salad with Lima Beans and Feta
  Jumbo Shrimp (3 oz.)   Snow Peas (1 cup)
  Baby Spinach (2 cups)   Lima Beans (¾ cup) GI = 32, GL = 9
  Black Olives (6)   Feta Cheese (1 TB.)
Vinaigrette Salad Dressing (2 TB.)

Lunch Glycemic Load: 9

Snack:

Real Ice Cream (⅓ cup) GI = 32, GL = 3
Lemonade (sugar-free, sweetened with Stevia)

Snack Glycemic Load: 3

Dinner:

Grilled Chicken Kabobs
  Mushrooms, Onion, Bell Pepper Chunks (1 cup)
  Chicken (3 oz.)
  Steamed Asparagus Tips (⅔ cup) GI = 10, GL = 1
  Black Beans and Corn (¾ cup) GI = 50, GL = 4
Cantaloupe (⅔ cup) GI = 65, GL = 6

Dinner Glycemic Load: 11

Snack:

Fresh Apple (1 medium) GI = 38, GL = 6   Almonds (6)

Snack Glycemic Load: 6

Total Glycemic Load for Friday: 61

Saturday:

Breakfast:
Poached Eggs
Zucchini/Tomato Stir-fry with Feta Cheese (1 oz.)
  Zucchini/Tomato, cooked (1 cup) GI = 10, GL = 1
Whole-grain Pumpernickel Bread (1 oz. slice) GI = 41, GL = 5
Honeydew Melon Cubes (1 cup) GI = 65, GL = 4

Breakfast Glycemic Load: 10

Snack:
Dates (4) GI = 50, GL = 10   Herbal Tea

Snack Glycemic Load: 10

Lunch:
Turkey and Pasta Salad with Feta Cheese
  Turkey (2 oz.)   Feta Cheese (1 oz.)
  Baby Greens with Sliced Onions and Chopped Basil (2 cups)
  Spiral Whole-wheat Pasta (⅓ cup, cooked al dente) GI = 44, GL = 7
  Green Olives
Lentil Soup
  Lentils, cooked (½ cup) GI = 29, GL = 4
  Onions/Carrots, chopped (¼ cup) GI = 10, GL = 1

Lunch Glycemic Load: 12

Snack:
Dried Peaches (4 halves) GI = 30, GL = 7   Almonds (6)
Herbal Tea

Snack Glycemic Load: 7

Dinner:
Poached Salmon with Rosemary (3 oz.)
Steamed Broccoli Spears Parmesan
  Broccoli (1 cup)   Parmesan Cheese (1 TB.)
Baked Yams (¾ cup) GI = 37, GL = 10
Yogurt, Plain Non-fat (½ cup) GI = 32, GL = 2

Dinner Glycemic Load: 12

Snack:
Pure Ice Cream (⅓ cup) GI = 32, GL = 3   Herbal Tea

Snack Glycemic Load: 3

Total Glycemic Load for Saturday: 54

Sunday:

Breakfast:

Steel-cut Oats and Bran with Raisins and Nuts

  Oats (¼ cup dry, cooks into ½ cup cooked) GI = 47, GL = 7

  Unprocessed Bran (¼ cup dry, cooks into ½ cup cooked) GI = 25, GL = 2

  Raisins (1 TB.) GI = 64, GL = 5

  Walnuts (2 large halves)

  Protein Powder or Nutritional Yeast (1 TB.) no carbs

Cottage Cheese and Pineapple

  2% Cottage Cheese (½ cup)   Pineapple, Unsweetened (⅓ cup) GI = 46, GL = 6

Breakfast Glycemic Load: 20

Snack:

Dried Apricots and Almonds

  Apricot (8 halves) GI = 30, GL = 4   Whole Almonds (6)

Snack Glycemic Load: 4

Lunch:

Lean Roast Beef Au Jus

Steamed Cabbage Confetti (2 cups)

  Tomatoes, chopped (½ cup) GI = 36, GL = 0

  Red Peppers, cut lengthwise (½ cup)

  Cabbage, shredded (1 cup)

Baked Butternut Squash with Cinnamon (1 cup) GI = 44, GL = 7

Whipped Peaches and Cream

  Canned Peaches, no sugar added (½ cup) GI = 48, GL = 7 and Cream (1 TB.)

  (whipped together)

Lunch Glycemic Load: 14

Snack:

Dark Chocolate (1 oz. square) GI = 48, GL = 8   Herbal Tea

Snack Glycemic Load: 8

Dinner:

Baked Chicken Breast (3 oz.)   Herb Brussels Sprouts Parmesan (1 cup)

New Red Potatoes with Skin (½ cup) GI = 76, GL = 11

Arugula and Baby Greens with Apple Slices

  Greens (2 cups)   Apple Slices (½ cup) GI = 38, GL = 6

  Salad Dressing (1 TB.)   Red Wine Vinegar (as desired)

Dinner Glycemic Load: 17

Snack:
Yogurt, Plain Non-fat (½ cup) GI = 32, GL = 2
Strawberries (⅔ cup) GI = 40, GL = 3

Snack Glycemic Load: 5

Total Glycemic Load for Sunday: 68

The Least You Need to Know

- ◆ Low-glycemic eating is the newest weight-loss eating plan.

- ◆ The glycemic index was developed to help people with diabetes manage blood sugar and insulin levels.

- ◆ By managing your insulin levels by eating low-glycemic, you can prevent fat storage and retain lean muscle mass as you lose weight.

Chapter 14

The Low-Carb Eating Plan

In This Chapter

- Enjoying low-carb meals for weight loss
- Eating nutrient-dense healthy foods
- Creating interesting meals

The ultra low-carb craze is over. Severely cutting carbs wasn't the answer to losing weight and keeping it off. Starvation-induction plans that put your body into ketosis are over and done with. But there's still plenty of value in eating low-carb meals.

With low-carb eating, you keep your energy high throughout the day while you jump-start your metabolism. With the menus in this chapter, you'll be eating enough carbs to lose weight, without severely restricting your food intake. You'll be able to eat with friends and family without apologizing for your odd and unusual food choices.

Eating Enough Carbs

Here's one low-carb eating program that keeps you out of starvation metabolism. That's important so that you lose weight steadily and keep your metabolism high. When a person doesn't eat enough carbs, their body loses muscle as well as fat. That can be a serious problem because your heart is a muscle the same as your thighs. Yes, perhaps you would like to lose some size in your thighs, but we know you don't want weight loss to mess with the strength of your heart or other vital body muscles.

The low-carb menus in this chapter give you about 100 grams of carbohydrates per day. From a dietary point of view, anything less than 180 grams of carbohydrates a day is low-carb. If you want to eat more than 100, you can increase the servings of bread or starch in the menus.

You need 80 grams per day to satisfy your brain's glucose needs, 30 grams per day to maintain your red blood cells, and 20 to 60 grams per day for healing wounds. To preserve muscle tissue, you need 100 to 180 grams of carbohydrates and adequate calories and protein. Otherwise, your body may break down muscle to build new glucose to meet your body's needs for fuel. And you need between 100 and 150 grams of carbs to keep you out of starvation metabolism.

Because your body needs carbs, the low-carb eating program doesn't have an induction program. An induction program is sometimes recommended to give you a jump-start on weight loss. It severely limits carbs for the first two weeks and isn't necessary for you to lose weight.

Most induction programs offer you less than 50 grams of carbs a day. Overall, induction programs simply aren't all that good for you, and you don't need to go on an induction program to lose weight.

Week 1 Menus for the Basic Low-Carb Eating Plan

Monday:

Breakfast:
Broiled Canadian Bacon (2 oz.) and
Tomato Parmesan, sliced (1 medium tomato and 2 tsp. Parmesan)
  on Corn Tortilla C = 5 or Low-Carb Flour Tortilla (1 small) C = 10
Fresh Peach Slices (1 peach) C = 15

Breakfast Carbs = 30

Snack:
Fresh Baby Carrots (⅓ cup) and Sugar Snap Peas (⅔ cup) C = 5
  with Toasted Peanuts (2 TB.) C = 2

Snack Carbs = 7

Lunch:
Spinach-Celery, Onion (3 cups chopped) Salad C = 12 with Red Grapes (¼ cup) C = 10
Grilled Salmon (3 oz.)
Vinaigrette Dressing (2 TB.)

Lunch Carbs = 22

Snack:
Fresh Pineapple Chunks (½ cup) C = 10
Herbal Tea

Snack Carbs = 10

Dinner:
Lemon-Pepper Chicken Breast (3 oz.)
Steamed Broccoli Spears (2 cups) C = 10
  with Feta Cheese (1 TB.)
Baked Yam (⅓ cup) C = 10
Butter (1 tsp.)

Dinner Carbs = 20

Snack:
Fresh Cantaloupe Slices (¾ cup) C = 10
Herbal Tea

Snack Carbs = 10

Total Carbs for Monday = 99

Tuesday:

Breakfast:
Whole-wheat Pita (small, ¾ oz.) or Low-Carb Tortilla C = 10 with Chicken (2 oz.)
  and Tomato, Onion, and Pepper (1 cup) C = 5 and Cheese (1 oz.)
Cucumber Spears (1 cup) C = 5
Fresh Whole Strawberries (1 cup) C = 10 with Unsweetened Whipped Cream (1 tsp.)

Breakfast Carbs = 30

Snack:
Avocado (⅛ large) and Celery (1 cup) C = 5

Snack Carbs = 5

Lunch:
Grilled Pork Tenderloin (3 oz.)
Fresh Steamed Green Beans (1 cup) C = 5 with Almond Slices (1 TB.)
Spinach/Romaine Greens (1 cup) with Vinaigrette Dressing (2 TB.)
Baked Winter Squash (½ cup) C = 15

Lunch Carbs = 20

Snack:
Pure Ice Cream (¼ cup) C = 7
Almonds (6) C = 1

Snack Carbs = 8

Dinner:
Beef Tenderloin (3 oz.) with Sun-dried Tomatoes (2 TB.) C = 5
Asparagus Spears (2 cups) C = 10
Wild Rice and Herbs (⅓ cup) C = 15
Mint Iced Tea with Lime

Dinner Carbs = 30

Snack:
Cantaloupe (¾ cup) C = 10
Chamomile Tea (iced or hot plain or with Stevia with FOS)

Snack Carbs = 10

Total Carbs for Tuesday = 103

Wednesday:

Breakfast:
Cheese (1 oz.) Pepper and Herb Omelet (1 egg, 2 egg whites)
Peppers and Herbs (½ cup) C = 2
Whole-wheat Low-carb Tortilla (6-in.) C = 10
Salsa (¼ cup) C = 3
Honeydew Melon Chunks (1 cup) C = 15

Breakfast Carbs = 30

Snack:
Crispy Broccoli and Cauliflower Flowerets (1 cup) C = 5
Oil and Vinegar Salad Dressing (1 TB.)

Snack Carbs = 5

Lunch:
Hearty Beef Vegetable Soup with
  Beef (2 oz.)
  Tomatoes, Carrots, Onions (2 cups) C = 10
  Navy or Pinto Beans (¼ cup) C = 7
Cantaloupe (½ cup) C = 7

Lunch Carbs = 24

Snack:
Dark Chocolate (¾ oz. square) or Veggies (2 cups) C = 10
Green Tea (decaf, iced, or hot)

Snack Carbs = 10

Dinner:
Barbequed Turkey (3 oz.)
Corn on the Cob (5-in.) C = 15
Summer Squash (1 cup) and Feta (1 tsp.) C = 5
Vinaigrette Coleslaw (1 cup) C = 5
Lemonade (sugar-free, sweetened with Stevia with FOS)

Dinner Carbs = 25

Snack:
Fresh Apple Slices (½ medium apple) C = 10
  with Peanut Butter (½ TB.) C = 2

Snack Carbs = 12

Total Carbs for Wednesday = 106

Thursday:

Breakfast:
Grilled Sirloin Strips (2 oz.)
Zucchini, Tomato, Onion (3 cups) C = 15 and Parmesan (2 TB.)
Fresh Apricots (3 small) C = 15

Breakfast Carbs = 30

Snack:
Cucumber Wedges (1 cup) C = 5 and Feta Cheese (1 TB.)

Snack Carbs = 5

Lunch:
Tuna Lettuce Wraps
 Tuna (3 oz.)
 Mayonnaise (1 tsp.)
 Mustard (½ tsp.)
 Romaine Leaves (4 large) C = 5
Spiced Whole Baby Beets, no sugar added (½ cup) C = 5
 with Sunflower Seeds (1 tsp.)
Fresh/Frozen Bing Cherries, no sugar added (½ cup) C = 10

Lunch Carbs = 20

Snack:
Pure Ice Cream (¼ cup) C = 7
Freshly Brewed Decaf, no sugar added

Snack Carbs = 7

Dinner:
Whole-grain Chicken Fajita
 Chicken, cooked, diced (2 oz.),
 Cheese (1 oz.)
 Peppers, Onions, cooked (1 cup) C = 10
 Low-Carbohydrate Whole-grain Tortilla (6-in.) C = 10
Salsa (¼ cup) C = 3
Celery, Carrot (1½ cups veggies), and Olive (6) Relish Tray C = 7

Dinner Carbs = 30

Snack:
Fresh Apple Slices (½ medium apple) C = 10   Walnuts (4)

Snack Carbs = 10

Total Carbs for Thursday = 102

Friday:

Breakfast:
Whole-wheat Pita with Cheese and Nuts
  Pita (¾ oz. or ⅓ small) or Low-carb Tortilla (1) C = 10
  Feta Cheese (1 oz.)
  Cottage Cheese (2 TB.) C = 1
  Almonds, slivered (4) C = 1
Fresh Whole Strawberries (1½ cups) C = 18

Breakfast Carbs = 30

Snack:
Grape Tomatoes (1 cup) C = 5

Snack Carbs = 5

Lunch:
Grilled Chicken (3 oz.)
Roasted Corn on the Cob (1–5-in.) C = 15
Fresh Seasoned Green Beans (½ cup) C = 3
Spinach Salad (1 cup) C = 2
Vinaigrette Dressing (1 TB.)

Lunch Carbs = 20

Snack:
Fresh Watermelon (¾ cup) C = 10
Herbal Tea

Snack Carbs = 10

Dinner:
Seafood Kabobs
  Large Shrimp (4), Scallops (4)
  Pea Pods and Onion, and Red Bell Peppers (2 cups) C = 10
  Pineapple Chunks (⅓ cup) C = 10
  Soy Sauce, Spices
Julienne Carrots, cooked (⅔ cup) C = 10

Dinner Carbs = 30

Snack:
Pure Ice Cream (¼ cup) C = 7
Herbal Tea

Snack Carbs = 7

Total Carbs for Friday = 102

Saturday:

Breakfast:
Steel-Cut Oats (½ cup cooked oats) C = 15 with Peaches and Cinnamon (⅓ cup peaches) C = 10
Cottage Cheese (½ cup) C = 4
Raw Almonds (12) C = 2

Breakfast Carbs = 31

Snack:
Sugar Snap Peas (½ cup) and Carrot Strips (½ cup) C = 5

Snack Carbs = 5

Lunch:
Spinach Salad with Chicken and Garbanzo Beans
  Spinach (2 cups) C = 10
  Chicken (3 oz.)
  Garbanzo Beans (⅓ cup) C = 10
  Ranch Salad Dressing (1 TB.)
  Red Wine Vinegar (unlimited)

Lunch Carbs = 20

Snack:
Dark Chocolate (¾ oz.) or Apple (½ medium) C = 10   Herbal Tea

Snack Carbs = 10

Dinner:
Grilled Tenderloin and Vegetable Kabobs
  Onions (½ cup) C = 3
  Whole Mushrooms (½ cup) C = 2
  Tomato Wedges (½ cup) C = 3
  Tenderloin Steak, cubed (3 oz.)
Black Beans with Green Onions (⅓ cup) C = 10
Berry Parfait
  Blueberries (⅓ cup) C = 5   Raspberries (⅓ cup) C = 5
  Whipped Cream (1 TB.)

Dinner Carbs = 28

Snack:
Fresh Bartlett Pear (½ small) C = 10   Herbal Tea

Snack Carbs = 10

Total Carbs for Saturday = 104

Sunday:

Breakfast:
Vegetable/Cheese Egg Omelet
  Raw Veggies, diced (1 cup) C = 5
  Grated Cheese (½ oz.)
  Egg (1) and Egg Whites (2)
Low-carb Whole-grain Toast (1 slice) C = 10
Fresh Grapefruit (½) C = 15
Butter (1 tsp.)

Breakfast Carbs = 30

Snack:
Edamame (Green Soybeans, lightly cooked, ½ cup) and Filberts C = 10
Herbal Tea

Snack Carbs = 10

Lunch:
Baked Cod
Steamed Asparagus Tips (1 cup) C = 5
Tomato/Onion Vinaigrette Salad (1 cup) C = 5
Whole-grain Pasta (¼ cup) C = 10

Lunch Carbs = 20

Snack:
Dates (2) C = 10
Herbal tea

Snack Carbs = 10

Dinner:
Taco Salad
  Cheese, shredded, (1 oz.)   Seasoned Turkey Strips (2 oz.)
  Avocado, chopped (⅛)
  Onion, Tomatoes, Peppers, Dark Greens (3 cups) C = 15
  Salsa (⅓ cup) C = 5
  Low-carb Whole-grain Bread, cut into triangles and baked until crispy (1 slice) C = 10

Dinner Carbs = 30

Snack:
Dried Apricots (4 halves) C = 7   Raw Almonds (12) C = 2

Snack Carbs = 9

Total Carbs for Sunday = 109

Week 2 Menus for the Basic Low-Carb Eating Plan

Monday:

Breakfast:
All-Bran Cereal (½ cup) C = 20
Milk, 1 percent (6 oz.) C = 9
Boiled Egg (2)

Breakfast Carbs = 29

Snack:
Grape Tomatoes (1 cup) C = 5

Snack Carbs = 5

Lunch:
Shrimp, Lima Bean, and Cashew Salad
  Shrimp (3 oz.)
  Romaine Lettuce, Onion, Celery (3 cups) C = 10
  Lima Beans (½ cup) C = 10
  Raw Cashews (12) C = 2
  Feta Cheese (½ oz.)
Vinaigrette Salad Dressing (2 TB.)

Lunch Carbs = 22

Snack:
Dark Chocolate (¾ oz.) or Raw Veggies (2 cups) C = 10
Herbal Tea

Snack Carbs = 10

Dinner:
Apricot-Chicken Stir Fry
  Chicken (3 oz.), Dried Apricot Halves, diced (6) C = 10
  Onion Slices and Red and Green Pepper Slices (3 cups) C = 15
  Brown Rice (2 TB.) C = 5
  Soy Sauce

Dinner Carbs = 30

Snack:
Peach Yogurt Parfait
  Sliced Peach (1 small fresh) C = 10

Snack Carbs = 10

Total Carbs for Monday = 106

Tuesday:

Breakfast:
Broiled Ham and Tomato with Cheddar
  Ham (2 oz.), Cheddar Cheese, shredded (1 oz.) on
  Tomato Slices, broiled (1 medium) C = 5
Black Beans with Fresh Tarragon (¼ cup) C = 7
Honeydew Melon Slices (¾ cup) C = 10

Breakfast Carbs = 22

Snack:
Sugar Snap Peas and Celery (1 cup) C = 5
Cashew Nuts (6) C = 1

Snack Carbs = 6

Lunch:
Turkey, Pecan, and Pear on Baby Greens
  Turkey, cut into strips (3 oz.), Pecan Halves (4), Fresh Pear, sliced (1) C = 20
  Baby Greens (2½ cups) C = 10
Vinaigrette Salad Dressing (2 TB.)

Lunch Carbs = 30

Snack:
Red Grapes (10 small) C = 10
Herbal Tea

Snack Carbs = 10

Dinner:
Spaghetti Squash with Sauce
  Squash (2 cups) C = 10
  Spaghetti Sauce (½ cup) C = 5
  Parmesan Cheese (1 oz.)
  Lean Ground Meat (2 oz.)
Fresh Blueberries (¾ cup) C = 15
  with Whipped Cream (1 TB.)

Dinner Carbs = 30

Snack:
Pure Ice Cream (¼ cup) C = 7
Herbal Tea

Snack Carbs = 7

Total Carbs for Tuesday = 105

Wednesday:

Breakfast:
Rolled Barley and Bran with Dried Apricots and Nuts
  Rolled Barley or Thick-cut Oats (¼ cup dry/½ cup cooked) C = 15
  Unprocessed Wheat Bran, added to oats (¼ cup dry) C = 5
  Dried Apricots, diced (6 halves) C = 10
  Almonds (12) C = 2
Grilled Ham Slices (2 oz.)
Herbal Tea

Breakfast Carbs = 32

Snack:
Carrot/Celery Sticks, raw (1 cup) C = 5

Snack Carbs = 5

Lunch:
Roasted Chicken and Vegetables
  Chicken (3 oz.)   Steamed Carrots, Fresh Green Beans, and Tomato (¾ cup) C = 4
Pea and Whole Pasta Salad
  Chopped Fresh Spinach and Onion (1 cup) C = 4   Peas (¼ cup) C = 6
  Pasta, cooked al dente (¼ cup) C = 10   Herbs and Spices
  Vinaigrette Dressing (2 TB.)

Lunch Carbs = 24

Snack:
Dark Chocolate (¾ oz. square) C = 10 or Sugar Snap Peas (1 cup) C = 5
Herbal Tea

Snack Carbs = 5

Dinner:
Haddock Fillet with Herbs (3 oz.)   Vinaigrette Coleslaw (1 cup) C = 5
Summer Squash, lightly cooked (1½ cups) C = 10
Spicy Sweet Potato Wedges (½ cup) C = 15

Dinner Carbs = 30

Snack:
Hot Cocoa (1 cup, sweetened with Stevia)
  1 percent or Skim Milk (6 oz.) C = 10   Unsweetened Cocoa Powder (1 tsp.)

Snack Carbs = 10

Total Carbs for Wednesday = 106

Thursday:

Breakfast:

Vegetable Egg Scramble with Cheese and Bacon Bits

  Egg (1) and Egg Whites (2)

  Onions, Tomatoes, Spinach, chopped and mixed with eggs (1 cup) C = 5

  Cheese, shredded on top of egg dish (½ oz.)

  Crispy Bacon, drained well, crumbled on egg dish (1 slice)

Strawberries (2 cups) C = 25

Breakfast Carbs = 30

Snack:

Broccoli and Cauliflower Flowerets (1 cup) C = 5   Ranch Dressing (1 TB.)

Snack Carbs = 5

Lunch:

Red Beans and Spinach with Turkey

  Spinach and Onions, chopped (3 cups) C = 10   Red Beans (¼ cup) C = 7

  Turkey, cut lengthways (2 oz.)   Feta Cheese, sprinkled on top (1 TB.)

Iced Tea

Lunch Carbs = 17

Snack:

Apple Slices (½ medium apple) C = 10   Filberts (10) C = 2

Snack Carbs = 12

Dinner:

Grilled Chicken Breast with Sun-dried Tomatoes

  Chicken (3 oz.)   Sun-dried Tomatoes (2 TB.) C = 5

Whole-grain Penne Rigate pasta, cooked al dente (¼ cup) C = 10

Pasta Sauce (¼ cup) C = 5

Sugar Snap Pea, Celery, and Sweet Red Pepper Salad (2 cups) C = 10

Green Olives (5)

Vinaigrette Dressing (2 TB.)

Dinner Carbs = 30

Snack:

Dark Chocolate (¾ oz. square) C = 10 or Pear (½ small) C = 10

Herbal Tea

Snack Carbs = 10

Total Carbs for Thursday = 104

Friday:

Breakfast:
Vegetable Egg Scramble and Low-carb Tortilla
  Egg (1) and Egg Whites (2)   Chopped Tomatoes, Onions, Spinach (1 cup) C = 5
  Low-carb Tortilla (1 small) C = 10   Salsa (¼ cup) C = 2
Red Beans and Spices (½ cup) C = 15

Breakfast Carbs = 32

Snack:
Watermelon, cubed (¾ cup) C = 10   Iced or Hot Herbal Tea

Snack Carbs = 10

Lunch:
Shrimp and Snow Pea, Spinach Salad with Lima Beans and Feta
  Jumbo Shrimp (3 oz.)   Snow Peas (1 cup) C = 5
  Baby Spinach (2 cups) C = 7   Lima Beans (½ cup) C = 10
  Black Olives (6)   Feta Cheese (1 TB.)
Vinaigrette Salad Dressing (2 TB.)

Lunch Carbs = 22

Snack:
Real Ice Cream (¼ cup) C = 7 or Raw Veggies (2 cups) C = 10
Lemonade (sugar-free, sweetened with Stevia)

Snack Carbs = 10

Dinner:
Grilled Chicken Kabobs
  Mushrooms, Onion, Bell Pepper Chunks (1 cup) C = 5
  Chicken (3 oz.)
  Steamed Asparagus Tips (½ cup) C = 3
  Black Beans and Corn (¼ cup) C = 7
Cantaloupe (½ cup) C = 7

Dinner Carbs = 22

Snack:
Fresh Apple (½ medium) C = 10
Almonds (6) C=1

Snack Carbs = 11

Total Carbs for Friday = 107

Saturday:

Breakfast:
Poached Eggs
Zucchini/Tomato Stir-fry with Feta Cheese
  Zucchini/Tomato, cooked (1 cup) C = 5   Feta Cheese (1 oz.)
Low-carb, Whole-grain Bread (1 oz. slice) C = 10
Honeydew Melon Cubes (1 cup) C = 15

Breakfast Carbs = 30

Snack:
Dates (2) C = 10   Herbal Tea

Snack Carbs = 10

Lunch:
Turkey and Pasta Salad with Feta Cheese
  Turkey (2 oz.)   Feta Cheese (1 oz.)
  Baby Greens with Sliced Onions and Chopped Basil (3 cups) C = 10
  Spiral Whole-wheat Pasta, cooked al dente (¼ cup) C = 10
  Green Olives

Lunch Carbs = 20

Snack:
Dried Peaches (2 Halves) C = 10
Almonds (6) C = 1
Herbal Tea

Snack Carbs = 11

Dinner:
Poached Salmon with Rosemary (3 oz.)
Steamed Broccoli Spears Parmesan
  Broccoli (1 cup) C = 5
  Parmesan Cheese (1 TB.)
Baked Yams (½ cup) C = 15
Yogurt, Plain Non-fat (½ cup) C = 10

Dinner Carbs = 30

Snack:
Pure Ice Cream (¼ cup) C = 7   Herbal Tea

Snack Carbs = 7

Total Carbs for Saturday = 108

Sunday:

Breakfast:
Steel-cut Oats and Bran with Raisins and Nuts
  Oats (¼ cup dry, cooks into ½ cup cooked) C = 15
  Unprocessed Bran, added to oats (¼ cup dry) C = 5
  Raisins (1 TB.) C = 7
  Walnuts (2 Large Halves)
  Protein Powder (without carbs)
Cottage Cheese, 2 percent (½ cup) C = 4

Breakfast Carbs = 31

Snack:
Dried Apricots and Almonds
  Apricot Halves (6) C = 10
  Whole Almonds (6) C = 1
Herbal Tea

Snack Carbs = 11

Lunch:
Lean Roast Beef Au Jus
Steamed Cabbage Confetti (2 cups)
  Tomatoes, chopped (½ cup) C = 3
  Red Peppers, cut lengthways (½ cup) C = 2
  Cabbage, shredded (1 cup) C = 5
Baked Butternut Squash with Cinnamon (¾ cup) C = 10

Lunch Carbs = 20

Snack:
Dark Chocolate (¾ oz. square) C = 10
Herbal Tea

Snack Carbs = 10

Dinner:
Baked Chicken Breast (3 oz.)
Herb Brussels Sprouts Parmesan (1 cup) C = 5
New Red Potatoes with Skin (¼ cup) C = 7

Arugula and Baby Greens with Apple Slices
  Greens (2 cups) C = 6
  Apple Slices (⅓ cup) C = 10
Salad Dressing (1 TB.)
Red Wine Vinegar (as desired)

Dinner Carbs = 28

Snack:
Strawberries (⅓ cup) C = 5
Herbal Tea

Snack Carbs = 5

Total Carbs for Sunday = 105

The Least You Need to Know

♦ Low-carb eating helps you lose weight by keeping your body's insulin levels low
  and fat-burning capacity high.

♦ You don't need to use an Induction phase to be successful losing weight with
  low-carb eating.

♦ Eat about 100 grams of carbohydrates a day to lose weight.

Chapter 15

The Low-Calorie Eating Plan

In This Chapter

- ◆ Counting calories
- ◆ A time-tested program
- ◆ Preparing healthy foods

For more than 50 years, people have used low-calorie eating to lose weight. Until about 20 years ago, experts thought that all foods were equal in their effect on weight gain. Not much research was done, if any, on how specific foods affected a person's weight gain or health.

Today, we know differently. The type of food you eat makes a big difference. But remember, 50 years ago, fast foods didn't exist. College students didn't survive on order-in pizza, and the large majority of families ate home-cooked meals together. The overall quality of the foods people ate was far better.

In this chapter, you'll find a low-calorie diet that includes wholesome foods and features the foods that keep your body from storing fat or depleting your lean muscle mass.

Your Daily Calorie Count and Nutritional Choices

The low-calorie menus in this chapter provide you with 1,500 calories a day. This amount will keep you out of starvation metabolism while you lose weight. Women can lose weight on this amount. If you are an active man, you can add 300 more calories to your menus every day.

You'll be eating top nutrition as you follow the menu plans. Whole grains, plenty of vegetables and fruit, and healthy meats and fish provide you with complete protein.

You won't find fast food or fluffy starches in your menu plans—those foods are seldom nutrient-dense. But if you want to pick up a main-dish salad from a fast-food restaurant on your way home from work, that could fit into your eating program.

> **Weighty Warning**
>
> Be sure to use your daily allotment of calories wisely. Don't eat them all at one meal. And don't save them up for one big hot-fudge sundae. Both strategies would put you into starvation metabolism, and the result could be that your body would store yet more fat. Instead, eat three meals a day plus snacks.

Is It a Fit?

A low-calorie meal plan could work well for you if …

◆ You already know how to count calories and are comfortable with doing so.

◆ You don't have health limitations such as diabetes, hypoglycemia, heart disease, autoimmune disorders, or high blood pressure.

◆ You don't have food sensitivities or allergies.

If you don't meet the preceding criteria, choose another eating program. Seriously consider the low-glycemic program.

Week 1 Menus for Low-Calorie Eating Plan

Monday:

Breakfast:
Broiled Canadian Bacon (2 oz.) Cal = 110 and
Tomato Parmesan
   Tomato, sliced (1 medium) Cal = 25   Parmesan (1 TB.) Cal = 25
   on Corn Tortilla (1 small) Cal = 80
Fresh Sugar Snap Peas (1 cup), Cal = 25

Breakfast calories = 265

Snack:
Fresh Peach Slices (1 peach) Cal = 60   Yogurt, Plain Low-fat (6 oz.) Cal = 90

Snack calories = 170

Lunch:
Spinach-Celery, chopped (3 cups) Cal = 75
Whole-grain Pasta (⅓ cup, cooked) Cal = 80
Salad with Red Grapes (⅓ cup) GI = 46, GL = 7 and
  Grilled Salmon (3 oz.) Cal = 165
  Vinaigrette Dressing, Low-fat (2 TB.) Cal = 45

Lunch calories = 425

Snack:
Fresh Pineapple Chunks (⅔ cup) Cal = 60 Dates (3) Cal = 60

Snack calories = 180

Dinner:
Baked Lemon-Pepper Chicken Breast (3 oz.) Cal = 105
Steamed Broccoli Spears (2 cups) Cal = 50
  with Feta Cheese (½ oz.) Cal = 40
Baked Yam (¾ cup) Cal = 120
Butter (1 tsp.) Cal = 40

Dinner calories = 395

Snack:
Fresh Cantaloupe Slices (1 cup) Cal = 60

Snack calories = 60

Total calories for Monday = 1,495

Tuesday:

Breakfast:
Whole-wheat Pita (1 oz.) Cal = 80 with Chicken Breast (2 oz.) Cal = 110 and
 Tomato, Onion, and Pepper (1 cup) Cal = 25 and Cheese (1 oz.) Cal = 100
Cucumber Spears (1 cup) Cal = 25
Fresh Whole Strawberries (1 cup) Cal = 60 with Whipped Cream (2 TB.) Cal = 20

Breakfast Calories = 340

Snack:
Avocado (¼ large) Cal = 90 and Celery (1 cup) Cal = 25

Snack Calories = 115

Lunch:
Grilled Pork Tenderloin (3 oz.) Cal = 165
Fresh Steamed Green Beans (1 cup) Cal = 25 with Almond Slices (1 TB.) Cal = 25
Spinach/Romaine Greens (2 cups) Cal = 35 with Vinaigrette Dressing, Low-fat
 (2 TB.) Cal = 45
Baked Winter Squash (¾ cup) Cal = 60 with
Apple Slices and Cinnamon (¼ cup) Cal = 40

Lunch calories = 395

Snack:
Pure Ice Cream (¼ cup) Cal = 75
Almonds (6) Cal = 45

Snack calories = 195

Dinner:
Beef Tenderloin (3 oz.) Cal = 165 with Sun-dried Tomatoes in Oil (2 TB.) Cal = 65
Asparagus Spears (2 cups) Cal = 50
Wild Rice and Herbs (½ cup) Cal = 100
Mint Iced Tea with Lime Cal = 0

Dinner calories = 380

Snack:
Cantaloupe (2 cups) Cal = 120
Chamomile Tea (iced or hot, plain or with Stevia with FOS)

Snack calories = 120

Total calories for Tuesday = 1,545

Wednesday:

Breakfast:
Cheese (1 oz.) Cal = 100 Pepper and Herb Omelet
  Egg (1) Cal = 80
  Egg Whites (2) Cal = 50
Whole-wheat Tortilla (6-in.) Cal = 80
Salsa (¼ cup) Cal = 20
Honeydew Melon Chunks (1 cup) Cal = 60

Breakfast calories = 390

Snack:
Crispy Broccoli and Cauliflower Flowerets (1 cup) Cal = 25

Snack calories = 25

Lunch:
Hearty Beef Vegetable Soup with
  Beef (3 oz.) Cal = 165
  Tomatoes, Carrots, Onions (1 cup) Cal = 50
  Navy or Pinto Beans (⅓ cup) Cal = 80
  Pearled Barley (⅓ cup) Cal = 80
Fresh Mango Slices (½ cup) Cal = 60 with Whipped Cream (2 TB.) Cal = 20

Lunch calories = 455

Snack:
Dark Chocolate (¾ oz.) Cal = 111   Green Tea (decaf, iced, or hot) Cal = 0

Snack calories = 111

Dinner:
Barbequed Turkey (3 oz.) Cal = 165
Corn on the Cob (5-in.) Cal = 80
Summer Squash (1 cup) Cal = 25 and Feta (1 TB.) Cal = 40
Vinaigrette Coleslaw, with Low-fat Dressing (1 cup) Cal = 55 with Cranberries
  (1 TB. dried) Cal = 25
Lemonade (sugar-free, sweetened with Stevia with FOS) Cal = 0
Butter (1 tsp.) Cal = 40

Dinner calories = 430

Snack:
Fresh Apple Slices (1 small apple) Cal = 60 with Peanut Butter (½ TB.) Cal = 45

Snack calories = 105

Total calories for Wednesday = 1,516

Thursday:

Breakfast:
Grilled Sirloin Strips (2 oz.) Cal = 110
Zucchini, Tomato, Onion (2 cups) Cal = 50 with Parmesan (1 TB.) Cal = 35
Hearty Whole-grain Bread (1 slice) Cal = 80
Fresh Apricots (3) Cal = 60

Breakfast calories = 335

Snack:
Cucumber Wedges (1 cup) Cal = 25 and Feta Cheese (1 TB.) Cal = 30

Snack calories = 55

Lunch:
Tuna Lettuce Wraps
  Tuna (3 oz.) Cal = 105   Mayonnaise (1 tsp.) Cal = 40
  Mustard (1 tsp.)   Romaine Leaves (4 large) Cal = 25
Spiced Whole Baby Beets, no sugar added (½ cup) Cal = 30
Long-grain Brown Rice (⅓ cup) Cal = 80 with Sunflower Seeds (1 tsp.) Cal = 10
Fresh/Frozen Bing Cherries (½ cup) Cal = 50 and
Plain, Non-fat Yogurt (6 oz.) Cal = 90

Lunch calories = 430

Snack:
Pure Ice Cream (¼ cup) Cal = 75   Freshly Brewed Decaf, no added sugar Cal = 0

Snack calories = 225

Dinner:
Whole-grain Chicken Fajita
  Diced Chicken Breast, cooked (2 oz.) Cal = 70
  Cheese (1 oz.) Cal = 100
  Peppers, Onions, cooked (½ cup) Cal = 25 and
  Whole-grain Flour Tortilla (one 6-in.) Cal = 80
Salsa (¼ cup) Cal = 20
Celery, Carrot (1½ cups veggies), and Olive (6) Relish Tray Cal = 75

Dinner calories = 370

Snack:
Fresh Apple Slices (1 large) Cal = 120   Walnuts (4) Cal = 40

Snack calories = 160

Total calories for Thursday = 1,500

Friday:

Breakfast:
Whole-wheat Pita with Cheese and Nuts
  Pita (1 oz. or ½ small) Cal = 80
  Feta Cheese (1 oz.) Cal = 75
  2 percent Cottage Cheese (½ cup) Cal = 90
  Almonds, chopped (6) Cal = 45
Fresh Whole Strawberries (2 cups) Cal = 100

Breakfast calories = 390

Snack:
Grape Tomatoes (1 cup) Cal = 35   Herbal Tea Cal = 0

Snack calories = 35

Lunch:
Grilled Chicken (3 oz.) Cal = 120
Roasted Corn on the Cob (1–5-in.) Cal = 80
Fresh Seasoned Green Beans (1 cup) Cal = 35
Spinach-Orange Salad
  Spinach, chopped (2 cups) Cal = 40 and Orange Slices (½ cup) Cal = 60
  Vinaigrette Dressing, Low-fat (2 TB.) Cal = 45
Butter (1 tsp.) Cal = 40

Lunch calories = 420

Snack:
Fresh Watermelon (1½ cups) 70   Herbal Tea

Snack calories = 70

Dinner:
Seafood Kabobs
  Large Shrimp (4), Scallops (4) Cal = 200
  Pea Pods, Onion, and Red Bell Peppers (2 cups) Cal = 50
  Pineapple Chunks (½ cup) Cal = 60
  Soy Sauce, Spices Cal = 0
Julienne Carrots (½ cup) Cal = 25 and Black Rice (⅓ cup) Cal = 80

Dinner calories = 390

Snack:
Pure Ice Cream (½ cup) Cal = 150   Herbal Tea Cal = 0

Snack calories = 150

Total calories for Friday = 1,480

Saturday:

Breakfast:
Steel-Cut Oats with Peaches and Cinnamon
  Oats, cooked (1 cup) Cal = 160   Unsweetened Peaches (½ cup) Cal = 60
2 percent Cottage Cheese (¾ cup) Cal = 135
Raw Almonds (6) Cal = 45

Breakfast calories = 400

Snack:
Sugar Snap Peas (1 cup) Cal = 25 and Carrot Strips (½ cup) Cal = 20

Snack calories = 45

Lunch:
Spinach Whole-grain Pasta Salad with Chicken and Garbanzo Beans
  Spinach, chopped (2 cups) Cal = 40
  Pasta, cooked al dente (⅓ cup) Cal = 80
  Chicken Breast (3 oz.) Cal = 105
  Garbanzo Beans (⅓ cup) Cal = 80
  Ranch Salad Dressing (2 TB.) Cal = 100
  Red Wine Vinegar (unlimited) Cal = 0

Lunch calories = 405

Snack:
Dark Chocolate (¾ oz.) Cal = 111
Fresh Apple (1 medium) Cal = 90   Herbal Tea Cal = 0

Snack calories = 201

Dinner:
Grilled Tenderloin and Vegetable Kabobs
  Onions (½ cup) Cal = 15   Whole Mushrooms (½ cup) Cal = 15
  Tomato Wedges (½ cup) Cal = 15   Tenderloin Steak, cubed (3 oz.) Cal = 165
Black Beans with Green Onions (½ cup) Cal = 80
Berry Parfait
  Blueberries (⅓ cup) Cal = 30   Raspberries (⅓ cup) Cal = 25
  Whipped Cream (2 TB.) Cal = 20

Dinner calories = 365

Snack:
Fresh Bartlett Pear (1 small) Cal = 100   Herbal Tea Cal = 0

Snack calories = 100

Total calories for Saturday = 1,516

Sunday:

Breakfast:

Vegetable/Cheese Egg Omelet
  Raw Veggies, diced (1 cup) Cal = 25   Grated Cheese (½ oz.) Cal = 50
  Egg (1) and Egg Whites (2) Cal = 130
Hearty Whole-grain Toast (1 slice) Cal = 80
Fresh Grapefruit (1 small, whole) Cal = 90
Butter (1 tsp.) Cal = 40

Breakfast calories = 415

Snack:

Edamame (Green Soybeans, lightly cooked, ½ cup) Cal = 50 and Filberts (10) Cal = 40
Herbal Tea Cal = 0

Snack calories = 90

Lunch:

Baked Cod (3 oz.) Cal = 105
Steamed Asparagus Tips (1 cup) Cal = 25
Tomato/Onion Vinaigrette (low-fat dressing) Salad (1 cup) Cal = 50
New Red Potatoes with Skin (5 oz.) Cal = 150
Butter (1 tsp.) Cal = 40

Lunch calories = 370

Snack:

Dates (6) Cal = 120   Herbal Tea

Snack calories = 120

Dinner:

Taco Salad
  Cheese, shredded, (1 oz.) Cal = 100
  Seasoned Turkey Breast Strips (2 oz.) Cal = 70
  Avocado, chopped (⅛) Cal = 45
  Onion, Tomatoes, Peppers, Dark Greens, chopped (3 cups) Cal = 75
  Salsa (¼ cup) Cal = 20
  Whole-grain Pita Bread, cut into triangles and baked until crispy (½ small) Cal = 80

Dinner calories = 390

Snack:

Dried Apricots (8 halves) Cal = 60   Raw Almonds (6) Cal = 45

Snack calories = 105

Total calories for Sunday = 1,490

Week 2 Menus for Low-Calorie Eating Plan

Monday:

Breakfast:
Museli (¾ cup) or All-Bran Cereal (1 cup) Cal = 160
Milk, 1 percent (8 oz.) Cal = 100
Banana Slices (1 medium) Cal = 90
Boiled Egg (1) Cal = 80

Breakfast calories = 430

Snack:
Grape Tomatoes (1 cup) Cal =35

Snack calorie = 35

Lunch:
Shrimp, Lima Bean, and Apple-Nut Salad
  Shrimp (3 oz.) Cal = 105
  Romaine Lettuce, Onion, Celery, chopped (3 cups) Cal = 75
  Apple Slices (1 medium apple) Cal = 90   Lima Beans (½ cup) Cal = 80
  Feta Cheese (½ oz.) Cal = 40   Raw Cashews (6) Cal = 45
Low-fat, Vinaigrette Salad Dressing (2 TB.) Cal = 45

Lunch calories = 480

Snack:
Dark chocolate (¾ oz.) Cal = 111   Herbal Tea Cal = 0

Snack calories = 111

Dinner:
Apricot-Chicken Stir Fry
  Chicken Breast (3 oz.) Cal = 105   Dried Apricot Halves, diced (8) Cal = 60
  Onion Slices and Red and Green Pepper Slices (2 cups) Cal = 50
  Brown Rice (⅓ cup) Cal = 80
Canola Oil (1 tsp.) Cal = 40

Dinner calories = 395

Snack:
Peach Yogurt Parfait
  Sliced Peach (1 fresh) Cal = 60
  Plain Nonfat Yogurt (½ cup) Cal=50

Snack calories = 110

Total calories for Monday = 1,561

Tuesday:

Breakfast:
Broiled Ham and Tomato with Cheddar
  Ham (2 oz.) Cal = 110
  Cheddar Cheese, shredded (1 oz.) Cal = 100 on Tomato Slices, broiled
    (1 medium tomato) Cal = 25
Black Beans with Fresh Tarragon (½ cup) Cal = 80
Honeydew Melon Slices (1 cup) Cal = 60

Breakfast total = 375

Snack:
Sugar Snap Peas and Celery (1 cup) Cal = 25
Cashew Nuts (6) Cal = 45

Snack total = 115

Lunch:
Turkey, Pecan and Pear on Baby Greens
  Turkey, cut into strips (3 oz.) Cal = 120
  Pecan Halves (4) Cal = 40
  Fresh Pear (1, sliced) Cal = 100
  Baby Greens (3 cups) Cal = 50
Coarsely Ground Whole-grain Toast (1 slice) Cal = 80
Low-fat Vinaigrette Salad Dressing (2 TB.) Cal = 45

Lunch total = 435

Snack:
Red Grapes (17 small) Cal = 60   Herbal Tea Cal = 0

Snack total = 60

Dinner:
Spaghetti Squash with Sauce
  Squash (2 cups) Cal = 60   Spaghetti Sauce (½ cup) Cal = 50
  Parmesan Cheese (1 oz.) Cal = 75   Lean Ground Meat, drained (2 oz.) Cal = 110
Fresh Blueberries (¾ cup) Cal = 65
  with Whipped Cream (2 TB.) Cal = 20

Dinner total = 360

Snack:
Pure Ice Cream (½ cup) Cal = 150   Herbal Tea Cal = 0

Snack total = 150

Total calories for Tuesday = 1,495

Wednesday:

Breakfast:

Rolled Barley and Bran with Dried Apricots and Nuts

  Rolled Barley or Thick-cut Oats (¼ cup dry/½ cup cooked) Cal = 80

  Unprocessed Wheat Bran (¼ cup dry, add to oats or barley) Cal = 45

  Dried Apricots (8 halves, diced) Cal = 60   Almonds (12) Cal = 90

Protein Fruit Shake

  Whey Protein Powder (2 TB.) (with no carbohydrates) Cal = 100

  Banana Slices (½ cup) Cal = 50   Strawberries (½ cup) Cal = 35

  Water and Ice (1 cup) Cal = 0   If desired, add Stevia to sweeten

Breakfast calories = 450

Snack:

Carrot Sticks, raw (2 cups) Cal = 60

Snack calories = 60

Lunch:

Roasted Chicken and Vegetables

  Chicken Breast (3 oz.) Cal = 105

  Carrots, Fresh Green Beans, and Tomato, cooked (1 cup) Cal = 50

Pea and Whole Pasta Salad

  Chopped Fresh Spinach and Onion (3 cups) Cal = 10

  Peas (½ cup) Cal = 70   Pasta, cooked al dente (⅓ cup) Cal = 80

  Herbs and Spices Cal = 0   Vinaigrette Dressing, Low-fat (2 TB.) Cal = 45

Lunch calories = 380

Snack:

Dark Chocolate (1 oz. square) Cal = 149   Herbal Tea Cal = 0

Snack calories = 149

Dinner:

Haddock Fillet with Herbs (3 oz.) Cal = 105

Vinaigrette Coleslaw, with Low-fat Dressing (1 cup) Cal = 55

Summer Squash, cooked (1 cup) Cal = 50

Spicy Sweet Potato Wedges (½ cup) Cal = 80   Butter (1 tsp.) Cal = 40

Dinner calories = 330

Snack:

Hot Cocoa (1 cup sweetened with Stevia) 1 percent or Skim Milk (1 cup) Cal = 100

  Unsweetened Cocoa Powder (1 tsp.) Cal = 10

Snack calories = 110

Total calories for Wednesday = 1,479

Thursday:

Breakfast:

Vegetable Egg Scramble with Cheese and Bacon Bits
  Egg (1) and Egg Whites (2) Cal = 130
  Onions, Tomatoes, and Spinach, chopped and mixed with eggs (1 cup) Cal = 25
  Cheese, shredded on top of egg dish (1 oz.) Cal = 100
  Crispy Bacon, drained well, crumbled on egg dish (1 slice) Cal = 50
Strawberries and Yogurt
  Strawberries (2 cups) Cal = 95   Yogurt, Non-fat Plain (1 cup) Cal = 110

Breakfast calories = 510

Snack:

Broccoli and Cauliflower Flowerets (1 cup), Cal = 25

Snack calories = 25

Lunch:

Red Beans, Spinach and Long-grain Brown Rice with Turkey
  Spinach and Onions, chopped (3 cups) Cal = 50   Brown Rice (⅓ cup) Cal = 80
  Red Beans (½ cup) Cal = 80   Feta Cheese (1 oz.) Cal = 75
  Turkey Breast, cut lengthways (2 oz.), Cal = 70
Iced Tea Cal = 0

Lunch calories = 355

Snack:

Apple Slices (1 medium) Cal = 90   Filberts or Peanuts (12) Cal = 90

Snack calories = 135

Dinner:

Grilled Chicken Breast with Sun-dried Tomatoes
  Chicken (3 oz.) Cal = 105   Sun-dried Tomatoes in Oil (2 TB.) Cal = 90
Whole-grain Penne Rigate (pasta) (⅓ cup, cooked al dente') Cal = 80
Pasta Sauce (¼ cup) Cal = 30
Sugar Snap Pea, Celery, and Sweet Red Pepper Salad (2 cups) Cal = 50
  Green Olives (6 large) Cal = 45
  Vinaigrette Dressing, Low-fat (2 TB.) Cal = 45

Dinner calories = 445

Snack:

Dates (3) Cal = 60   Herbal Tea Cal = 0

Snack calories = 60

Total calories for Thursday = 1,490

Friday:

Breakfast:

Vegetable Egg Scramble and Corn Tortilla
  Egg (1) and Egg Whites (2) Cal = 130
  Chopped Tomatoes, Onions, and Spinach (1 cup) Cal = 25
  Corn Tortilla (1 small) Cal = 80
  Salsa (¼ cup) Cal = 20
Red Beans and Spices (½ cup) Cal = 80
Kiwi Slices (½ cup) Cal = 60

Breakfast calories = 395

Snack:

Watermelon, cubed (1 cup) Cal = 50   Iced or Hot Herbal Tea Cal = 0

Snack calories = 50

Lunch:

Shrimp and Snow Pea, Spinach Salad with Lima Beans and Feta
  Jumbo Shrimp (3 oz.) Cal = 105   Snow Peas (1 cup) Cal = 25
  Baby Spinach (3 cups) Cal = 10   Lima Beans (¾ cup) Cal = 80
  Black Olives (6) Cal = 45   Feta Cheese (1 oz.) Cal = 75
Vinaigrette Salad Dressing, Low-fat (2 TB.) Cal = 45

Lunch calories = 405

Snack:

Real Ice Cream (⅓ cup) Cal = 90
Lemonade (sugar-free, sweetened with Stevia) Cal = 0

Snack calories = 90

Dinner:

Grilled Chicken Kabobs
  Mushrooms, Onion, Bell Pepper Chunks (1 cup) Cal = 25
  Chicken Breast (3 oz.) Cal = 105
  Steamed Asparagus Tips (1 cup) Cal = 25
  Black Beans and Corn (¾ cup) Cal = 120
Cantaloupe (1 cup) Cal = 60

Dinner calories = 335

Snack:

Fresh Apple (1 medium) Cal = 90
Almonds (12) Cal = 90

Snack calories = 180

Total calories for Friday = 1,455

Saturday:

Breakfast:
Poached Eggs (2) Cal = 160
Zucchini/Tomato Stir-Fry with Feta Cheese
    Zucchini/Tomato, cooked (1 cup) Cal = 50   Feta Cheese (1 oz.), Cal = 75
Whole-grain Pumpernickel Bread (1 oz. slice) Cal = 80
Honeydew Melon Cubes (1 cup) Cal = 60
Butter (1 tsp.) Cal = 45

Breakfast calories = 470

Snack:
Dates (4) Cal = 80   Herbal Tea Cal = 0

Snack calories = 80

Lunch:
Turkey and Pasta Salad with Feta Cheese
    Turkey Breast (2 oz.) Cal = 70   Feta Cheese (1 oz.) Cal = 75
    Baby Greens with Sliced Onions and Chopped Basil (3 cups) Cal = 10
    Spiral Whole-wheat Pasta (⅓ cup, cooked al dente) Cal = 80
    Green Olives (6) Cal = 50
Lentil Soup
    Lentils, cooked (½ cup) Cal = 80   Onions/Carrots, chopped (¼ cup) Cal = 10

Lunch calories = 395

Snack:
Dried Peaches (4 halves) Cal = 30
Almonds (6) Cal = 45
Herbal Tea

Snack calories = 75

Dinner:
Poached Salmon with Rosemary (3 oz.) Cal = 165
Steamed Broccoli Spears, Parmesan
    Broccoli (1 cup) Cal = 25   Parmesan Cheese (1 TB.) Cal = 30
Baked Yams (¾ cup) Cal = 120
Yogurt, Plain Non-fat (6 oz. cup) Cal = 90

Dinner calories = 430

Snack:
Pure Ice Cream (¼ cup) Cal = 75   Herbal tea Cal = 0

Snack calories = 90

Total calories for Saturday = 1,525

Sunday:

Breakfast:
Steel-cut Oats and Bran with Raisins and Nuts
  Oats (¼ cup dry cooks into ½ cup cooked) Cal = 80
  Unprocessed Bran, cooked into the oats (¼ cup dry) Cal = 25
  Raisins (1 TB.) Cal = 30
  Walnuts (2 Large Halves) Cal = 20
  Protein Powder or Nutritional Yeast (1 TB. without carbs) Cal = 50
Cottage Cheese and Pineapple
  2 percent Cottage Cheese (½ cup) Cal = 90
  Pineapple, Unsweetened (⅓ cup) Cal = 50

Breakfast calories = 345

Snack:
Dried Apricots and Almonds
  Apricot Halves (8) Cal = 60
  Whole Almonds (6) Cal = 45

Snack calories = 105

Lunch:
Lean Roast Beef (3 oz.) Au Jus Cal = 165
Steamed Cabbage Confetti (2 cups) Cal = 50
  Tomatoes, chopped (½ cup) Cal = 15
  Red Peppers, cut lengthways (½ cup) Cal = 10
  Cabbage, shredded (1 cup) Cal = 25
Baked Butternut Squash with Cinnamon (1 cup) Cal = 80
Whipped Peaches and Cream
  Peaches, canned, no sugar (½ cup) Cal = 60
  Whipped Cream (2 TB.) Cal = 20

Lunch calories = 425

Snack:
Dark Chocolate (¾ oz. square) Cal = 111
Herbal Tea Cal = 0

Snack calories = 111

Dinner:
Baked Chicken Breast (3 oz.) Cal = 105
Herb Brussel Sprouts (1 cup) Cal = 25 with Parmesan (½ oz.) Cal = 40
New Red Potatoes with Skin (½ cup) Cal = 80
Arugula and Baby Greens with Apple Slices
  Greens (3 cups) Cal = 10
  Apple Slices (½ cup) Cal = 60
Ranch Salad Dressing (1 TB.) Cal = 45
Red Wine Vinegar (as desired) Cal = 0

Dinner calories = 385

Snack:
Yogurt, Plain Non-fat (6 oz.) Cal = 90
Strawberries (½ cup) Cal = 30

Snack calories = 120

Total calories for Sunday = 1,491

The Least You Need to Know

- Low-calorie eating plans have been used for more than 50 years for weight loss.

- You can eat about 1,500 calories a day to lose weight.

- If you're very active, you may be able to add an additional 300 calories a day and still lose weight.

Chapter 16

The Low-Fat Eating Plan

In This Chapter

- When eating low-fat is recommended
- Keeping your fat intake between 20 and 30 percent
- Eating wholesome low-fat foods
- Avoiding low-fat mistakes

Extreme low-fat diets were all the rage more than 10 years ago when researchers found that people with heart disease and high cholesterol had a build-up of fat in their arteries. The underlying assumption was that dietary fat caused clogged arteries.

Fast forward to the present. Eating high amounts of dietary fat is only one factor in heart disease. Some other factors are a high intake of starchy foods, high insulin and cortisol levels in the blood, lack of exercise, and a lack of Essential Fatty Acids in a person's diet.

Today, many medical practitioners and dietitians recommend eating low-fat, so this chapter gives you some ideas of what to eat if you need to eat low-fat meals.

The Best Amount

Gone are the days when diet pals vied for the honor of eating the lowest amount of fat in their diets. Sure, they lost weight for a while, but then their bodies refused to release more fat. In fact, their body was hoarding fat. Why? Because everyone needs a certain amount of dietary fat to be healthy. And everyone needs essential fatty acids to lose weight and release fat.

Dietary fat adds satiation to the feel of a meal. When you eat the right amount of fat at each meal, you'll push your chair away with a feeling of completion. Because you'll be satisfied, you won't be noshing the whole rest of the day.

The American Heart Association recommends eating 30 percent or less of your calories in fat daily. In the menus that follow, we've given you 42 milligrams of fat per day.

Fat Doesn't Make You Fat

One highly educated friend believed that if she ate any dietary fat, it went instantly into the fat stores on her hips and thighs. Her thinking is still popular today, but her thinking is an urban myth.

When you eat fat, it goes first to the stomach, where it is digested and then to the intestinal tract, where it is absorbed and assimilated by the body. Only if you eat too much food is the food you eat stored as fat. And, by the way, any food you overeat is stored as fat—cereal, steak, sour cream, and even vegetables.

Add in Your EFAs

The menus that follow allow for you to take one tablespoon of Essential Fatty Acids daily as part of your fat intake. Be sure to take them. They make you thin.

Yes, research has shown that when you take Essential Fatty Acids, your body more readily releases fat. When you eat about 20-30 percent of your calories in dietary fat, your body also releases stored fat more easily.

About the Menus

The following menus contain between 36 and 42 grams of fat per day, or about 20 to 25 percent of the calories from fat. This is based on eating 1500 calories per day. The foods recommended are mostly regular foods, as opposed to low-fat foods, which you eat in smaller portions.

In the menus that follow, the 42 grams of fat per day come from …

Weighty Warning

Beware of some packaged and processed foods labeled "low-fat." Often these contain lots of high-glycemic starches and sugars that can lift your blood sugar levels and cause your body to store more fat. An exception is low-fat dairy products and some salad dressings. Check labels before you purchase.

- ◆ Lean to moderately lean proteins such as chicken, fish, beef, pork, and cottage cheese and small amounts of proteins higher in fat such as cheese and bacon.

- ◆ Fats that are added to food, which include butter, salad dressing, vegetable oils, and peanut butter.

- ◆ Nuts and seeds, including almonds, peanuts, cashews, pecans, walnuts, and sesame seeds.

- ◆ Some grain and legume foods, like tortillas, soybeans, and whole-grain breads.

The combinations of fats give you a healthy fatty-acid balance of monounsaturated, polyunsaturated, and saturated fats.

Although you'll be eating based on these menus, be sure that you always honor your body's needs for food. Eat 0–5. If you have more food remaining in your meal, but you are already at a 5, stop eating. Overeating will always make you overweight.

Week 1 Menus for Low-Fat Eating Plan

Monday:

Breakfast:
Broiled Canadian Bacon (2 oz.) F = 6 and
Tomato Parmesan F = 3
  Sliced Tomato (1 medium)
  Parmesan (1 oz.)
Shredded Spinach (1 cup) on Corn Tortilla (1 small) F = 2
Fresh Peach Slices (1 peach)
Yogurt, Plain Fat-free (6 oz.)

Breakfast Fat Grams = 11

Snack:
Fresh Apple (1) with Toasted Peanuts (10) F = 5

Snack Fat Grams = 5

Lunch:
Spinach-Celery, chopped (2 cups)
Whole-grain Pasta, cooked (⅓ cup) F = 1
Salad with Red Grapes (⅓ cup) and Grilled Salmon (3 oz.) F = 9
Vinaigrette Dressing, Low-fat (2 TB.) F = 5

Lunch Fat Grams = 14

Snack:
Fresh Pineapple Chunks (⅔ cup)

Snack Fat Grams = 0

Dinner:
Lemon-Pepper Chicken Breast (3 oz.) F = 3
Steamed Broccoli Spears (2 cups)
Baked Yam (1 cup)
Butter (1 tsp.) F = 5

Dinner Fat Grams = 8

Snack:
Fresh Cantaloupe Slices (1 cup)

Snack Fat Grams = 0

Total Fat Grams for Monday = 38

Tuesday:

Breakfast:
Whole-wheat Pita (1 oz.) F = 1
Chicken Breast (2 oz.) F = 2 and Tomato, Onion, Pepper, and Cheese (1 oz.) F = 8
Cucumber Spears (1 cup)
Fresh Whole Strawberries (1 cup)

Breakfast Fat Grams = 11

Snack:
Avocado (⅛ large) F = 5 and Celery (1 cup)

Snack Fat Grams = 5

Lunch:
Grilled Pork Tenderloin (3 oz.) F = 9
Fresh Steamed Green Beans (1 cup)

Spinach/Romaine Greens (1 cup) with Vinaigrette Dressing, Low-fat (2 TB.) F = 5
Baked Winter Squash (¾ cup) with Apple Slices and Cinnamon (½ cup)

Lunch Fat Grams = 14

Snack:
Dates (3)
Herbal Tea

Snack Fat Grams = 0

Dinner:
Beef Tenderloin (3 oz.) F = 9 with Sun-dried Tomatoes in Oil (1–2 TB.) F = 3
Asparagus Spears (1 cup)
Wild Rice and Herbs (⅓ cup)
Papaya Slices (½ cup)
Mint Iced Tea with Lime

Meal Fat Grams = 12

Snack:
Plain, Non-fat Yogurt (6 oz.)
Chamomile Tea (iced or hot, plain or with Stevia with FOS)

Snack Fat Grams = 0

Total Fat Grams for Tuesday = 42

Wednesday:

Breakfast:
Cheese (1 oz.) F = 9
Pepper and Herb Omelet
  Egg (1) and Egg Whites (2) F = 5
  Green Peppers and Onions, chopped (1 cup)
Whole-wheat Tortilla (6-in.) F = 2
Salsa (½ cup)
Honeydew Melon Chunks (1 cup) GI = 65, GL = 4

Breakfast Fat Grams = 16

Snack:
Crispy Broccoli and Cauliflower Flowerets and Carrot Sticks (1 cup)

Snack Fat Grams = 0

Lunch:
Hearty Beef Vegetable Soup with
  Beef (2 oz.) F = 6   Tomatoes, Carrots, Onions (1 cup)
  Navy or Pinto Beans (⅓ cup)   Pearled Barley (¼ cup)
Fresh Mango Slices (½ cup)

Lunch Fat Grams = 6

Snack:
Cantaloupe (1 cup)
Green Tea (decaf, iced, or hot)

Snack Fat Grams = 0

Dinner:
Barbequed Turkey Breast (3 oz.) F = 3
Corn on the Cob (5-in.) and Feta Cheese (½ oz.) F = 2
Vinaigrette Coleslaw (1 cup) with Low-fat Vinaigrette Dressing (2 TB.) F = 5 and
  Cranberries, dried (2 TB.)
Butter (1 tsp.) F = 5
Lemonade (sugar-free, sweetened with Stevia with FOS)

Dinner Fat Grams = 15

Snack:
Fresh Apple Slices (1 small apple) GI = 38, GL = 6 with Peanut Butter (½ TB.) F = 5

Snack Fat Grams = 5

Total Fat Grams for Wednesday = 42

Thursday:

Breakfast:
Grilled Sirloin Strips (2 oz.) F = 6
Zucchini, Tomato, Onion (2 cups) Parmesan (½ oz.) F = 1
Hearty Whole-grain Bread (1 slice) F = 1
Fresh Apricots (3)
Peanut Butter or other nut spread (½ TB.) F = 5

Breakfast Fat Grams = 13

Snack:
Cucumber Wedges (2 cups)

Snack Fat Grams = 0

Lunch:
Tuna Lettuce Wraps
  Tuna (3 oz.) F = 2   Mayonnaise (1 tsp.) F = 5
  Mustard (½ tsp.) and   Romaine Leaves (4 large)
Spiced Whole Baby Beets, no sugar added (½ cup)
Long-grain Brown Rice (⅓ cup)
Fresh/Frozen Bing Cherries (¼ cup)
Plain Non-fat Yogurt (4 oz.)

Lunch Fat Grams = 7

Snack:
Dates (3)   Freshly Brewed Decaf (no added sugar)

Snack Fat Grams = 0

Dinner:
Whole-grain Chicken Fajita
  Diced Chicken Breast, cooked (2 oz.) F = 2   Cheese (1 oz.) F = 8
  Peppers, Onions, cooked (½ cup) and Whole-grain Flour Tortilla (one 6-inch) F = 2
Avocado (⅛ medium) F = 5
Celery, Carrot, Cucumber Relish Tray (1 cup veggies)
Fresh Peach (1)

Meal Fat Grams = 17

Snack:
Fresh Apple Slices (½ cup)

Snack Fat Grams = 0

Total Fat Grams for Thursday = 37

Friday:

Breakfast:
Whole-wheat Pita with Cheese and Nuts
  Pita (1 oz. or ½ small) F = 1
  Feta Cheese (½ oz.) F = 2
  2 percent Cottage Cheese (½ cup) F = 2
  Almonds (6, chopped) F = 5
Fresh Whole Strawberries (1 cup)

Breakfast Fat Grams = 10

Snack:
Grape Tomatoes and Celery Sticks (1 cup)

Snack Fat Grams = 0

Lunch:
Grilled Chicken Breast (3 oz.) F = 3
Roasted Corn on the Cob (1–5-in.)
Fresh Seasoned Green Beans (1 cup)
Spinach-Orange Salad (1 cup spinach and ½ cup orange slices)
Vinaigrette Dressing, Low-fat (2 TB.) F = 5
Butter (1 tsp.) F = 5

Lunch Fat Grams = 13

Snack:
Fresh Watermelon (1 cup)   Herbal Tea

Snack Fat Grams = 0

Dinner:
Seafood Kabobs
  Large Shrimp and Scallops (3 oz.) F = 2
  Pea Pods, Onion, and Red Bell Peppers (½ cup)
  Pineapple Chunks (½ cup)
  Soy Sauce, Spices, Canola Oil (1 tsp.) F = 5
Julienne Carrots (½ cup) and Black Rice (⅓ cup)
Almond Slices (2 TB.) F = 5

Dinner Fat Grams = 12

Snack:
Pure Ice Cream (⅓ cup) F = 7   Herbal Tea

Snack Fat Grams = 7

Total Fat Grams for Friday = 42

Saturday:

Breakfast:

Steel-Cut Oats with Peaches and Cinnamon
  Oats (½ cup cooked or ¼ cup dry)
  Raisins (2 TB.)   Peaches (½ cup)
2 percent Cottage Cheese (¾ cup) F = 3
Raw Almonds (12) F = 10

Breakfast Fat Grams = 13

Snack:

Sugar Snap Peas (1 cup) and Carrot Strips (1 cup)

Snack Fat Grams = 0

Lunch:

Spinach Whole-grain Pasta Salad with Chicken and Garbanzo Beans
  Spinach (2 cups)   Pasta, cooked al dente (⅓ cup) F = 1
  Chicken Breast (3 oz.) F = 3   Garbanzo Beans (⅓ cup) F = 1
  Ranch Salad Dressing (2 TB.) F = 10   Red Wine Vinegar (unlimited)
Dried Apricots (8 halves)

Lunch Fat Grams = 15

Snack:

Fresh Apple (1)   Herbal Tea

Snack Fat Grams = 0

Dinner:

Grilled Tenderloin and Vegetable Kabobs
  Onions (½ cup)   Whole Mushrooms (½ cup)
  Tomato Wedges (½ cup)   Tenderloin Steak (3 oz. cubed) F = 9
Black Beans with Green Onions (½ cup)
Berry Parfait
  Blueberries (½ cup)
  Raspberries (½ cup)
  Whipped Cream (1 TB.) F = 5

Meal Fat Grams = 14

Snack:

Fresh Bartlett Pear (1 small)   Herbal Tea

Snack Fat Grams = 0

Total Fat Grams for Saturday = 42

Sunday:

Breakfast:
Vegetable/Cheese Egg Omelet
  Raw Veggies, diced (1 cup)   Grated Cheese (¼ oz.) F = 2
  Egg (1) and Egg Whites (2) F = 5
Hearty Whole-grain Toast (1 slice) F = 1
Fresh Grapefruit (1 small whole)
Butter (1 tsp.) F = 5

Breakfast Fat Grams = 13

Snack:
Edamame (Green Soybeans, lightly cooked, ½ cup) F = 4
Herbal Tea

Snack Fat Grams = 4

Lunch:
Baked Cod (3 oz.) F = 3
Steamed Asparagus Tips (1 cup)
Tomato/Onion Vinaigrette Salad (1 cup) with Vinaigrette Salad dressing (2 TB.) F = 5
New Red Potatoes with Skin (6 oz.)
Peach (1 fresh)

Lunch Fat Grams = 8

Snack:
Dates (3)   Herbal Tea

Snack Fat Grams = 0

Dinner:
Taco Salad
  Cheese, shredded, (1 oz.) F = 5
  Seasoned Turkey Strips (2 oz.) F = 2
  Avocado, chopped (⅛) F = 5
  Onion, Tomatoes, Peppers, Dark Greens (3 cups)
  Salsa (¼ cup)
  Whole-grain Pita Bread, cut into triangles and baked until crispy (½ small) F = 1

Dinner Fat Grams = 13

Snack:
Dried Apricots (8 halves)   Raw Almonds (4) F = 3

Snack Fat Grams = 3

Total Fat Grams for Sunday = 41

Week 2 Menus for Low-Fat Eating Plan

Monday:

Breakfast:
All-Bran Cereal (1 cup) F = 2
Milk, skim (8 oz.)
Banana Slices (1 small banana)
Boiled Egg (1) F = 5
Raw Almonds (6) F = 5
Breakfast Fat Grams = 12

Snack:
Grape Tomatoes (2 cups)
Snack Fat Grams = 0

Lunch:
Shrimp, Lima Bean, and Apple-Nut Salad
  Shrimp (3 oz.) F = 2   Romaine Lettuce, Onion, Celery (3 cups)
  Apple Slices (1 large apple)   Lima Beans (⅔ cup)
  Raw Cashews (6) F = 5   Feta Cheese (½ oz.) F = 4
  Vinaigrette Salad Dressing, Low-fat (2 TB.) F = 5
Lunch Fat Grams = 16

Snack:
Orange, fresh (1)   Herbal Tea
Snack Fat Grams = 0

Dinner:
Apricot-Chicken Stir Fry
  Chicken Breast (3 oz.) F = 3 Dried Apricot Halves (8, diced)
  Cashews (12) F = 10   Onion Slices and Red and Green Pepper Slices (2 cups)
  Brown Rice (⅓ cup)
Meal Fat Grams = 13

Snack:
Peach Yogurt Parfait
  Sliced Peaches (1 fresh)   Plain Non-fat Yogurt (½ cup)
Snack Fat Grams = 0

Total Fat Grams for Monday = 41

Tuesday:

Breakfast:

Broiled Ham and Tomato with Cheddar

  Ham (2 oz.) F = 6

  Cheddar Cheese (½ oz.) F = 4 shredded on Tomato Slices, broiled (1 medium tomato)

Spinach, chopped (1 cup)

Black Beans with Fresh Tarragon (½ cup) F = 1

Honeydew Melon Slices (2 cups)

Breakfast Fat Grams = 11

Snack:

Sugar Snap Peas and Celery (2 cups)   Cashew Nuts (6) F = 5

Snack Fat Grams = 5

Lunch:

Turkey, Pecan and Pear on Baby Greens

  Turkey Breast, cut into strips (3 oz.) F = 3   Pecan Halves (5) F = 5

  Fresh Pear, sliced (1)   Baby Greens (2 cups)

Coarsely Ground Whole-grain Toast (1 slice) F = 1

Vinaigrette Salad Dressing, Low-fat (2 TB.) F = 5

Lunch Fat Grams = 14

Snack:

Red Grapes (17 small)   Herbal Tea

Snack Fat Grams = 0

Dinner:

Spaghetti Squash with Sauce

  Squash (2 cups)

  Spaghetti Sauce (½ cup) F = 1

  Parmesan Cheese (½ oz.) F = 1

  Lean Ground Meat (3 oz.) F = 9

Whole-grain, Stone-ground Dinner Roll F = 1

Fresh Blueberries and Peach Slices (1 cup)

Dinner Fat Grams = 12

Snack:

Fresh Strawberries (1 cup)

Herbal Tea

Snack Fat Grams = 0

Total Fat Grams for Tuesday = 42

Wednesday:

Breakfast:
Rolled Barley and Bran with Dried Apricots and Nuts
  Rolled Barley or Thick-cut Oats (¼ cup dry/½ cup cooked)
  Unprocessed Wheat Bran (¼ cup dry/½ cup cooked)
  Dried Apricots (8 halves, diced)   Almonds (12) F = 10
Protein Fruit Shake
  Whey Protein Powder (2 TB.) (with no carbohydrates or fat)
  Banana Slices (½ cup)   Strawberries (½ cup)
  Plain Yogurt or Skim Milk (½ cup) and Ice   If desired, Stevia to sweeten
Breakfast Fat Grams = 10

Snack:
Carrot-Celery Sticks, raw (2 cups)   Herbal Tea
Snack Fat Grams = 0

Lunch:
Roasted Chicken and Vegetables
  Chicken (3 oz.) F = 3   Carrots, Fresh Green Beans, and Tomato, cooked (1 cup)
Pea and Whole Pasta Salad
  Chopped Fresh Spinach and Onion (1 cup)
  Peas (¼ cup)   Cheese (½ oz.) F = 4
  Pasta, cooked al dente (⅓ cup) F = 1   Herbs and Spices
  Vinaigrette Dressing, Low-fat (2 TB.) F = 5
Lunch Fat Grams = 13

Snack:
Dark Chocolate (1 oz. square) F = 9   Herbal Tea
Snack Fat Grams = 9

Dinner:
Haddock Fillet with Herbs (3 oz.) F = 3
Vinaigrette Coleslaw (1 cup) with Low-fat Vinaigrette Dressing F = 5
Summer Squash, cooked (1 cup)   Spicy Sweet Potato Wedges (6 oz.)
Meal Fat Grams = 8

Snack:
Hot Cocoa (1 cup sweetened with Stevia)
  Skim Milk (1 cup)   Unsweetened Cocoa Powder (1 tsp.) F = 1
Snack Fat Grams = 1

Total Fat Grams for Wednesday = 41

Thursday:

Breakfast:
Vegetable Egg Scramble with Cheese and Bacon Bits
  Egg (1) and Egg Whites (2) F = 5
  Onions, Tomatoes, Spinach, (2 cups, chopped) and Red Beans, mixed with eggs
  (⅓ cup) F = 1
  Cheese, shredded on top of egg dish (½ oz.) F = 4
  Crispy Bacon, drained well, crumbled on egg dish (1 slice) F = 5 ()
Strawberries and Yogurt
  Strawberries (1 cup)   Yogurt, Non-fat Plain (6 oz.)
Breakfast Fat Grams = 15

Snack:
Broccoli and Cauliflower Flowerets (1 cup)
Snack Fat Grams = 0

Lunch:
Black Beans, Spinach and Long-Grain Brown Rice with Turkey
  Spinach and Onions, chopped (2 cups)
  Black Beans (½ cup)   Brown Rice (⅓ cup)
  Turkey Breast, cut lengthways (3 oz.) F = 3
  Feta Cheese, sprinkled on top (½ oz.) F = 4
Iced Tea
Lunch Fat Grams = 7

Snack:
Apple Slices (1 small apple)
Snack Fat Grams = 0

Dinner:
Grilled Chicken Breast with Sun-dried Tomatoes
  Chicken (3 oz.) F = 3   Sun-dried Tomatoes in Oil (2 TB.) F = 5
Whole-grain Penne Rigate (pasta) (⅔ cup, cooked al dente) F = 1
Pasta Sauce (½ cup) F = 1
Sugar Snap Pea, Celery, and Sweet Red Pepper Salad (2 cups)
Green Olives (6) F = 5   Vinaigrette Dressing, Low-fat (2 TB.) F = 5
Dinner Fat Grams = 20

Snack:
Dates (3)   Herbal Tea
Snack Fat Grams = 0

Total Fat Grams for Thursday = 42

Friday:

Breakfast:
Vegetable Egg Scramble and Corn Tortilla
  Egg (1) and Egg Whites (2) F = 5
  Tomatoes, Onions, Spinach, chopped (1 cup)
  Corn Tortilla (1 small) F = 2
  Salsa (½ cup)
Red Beans and Spices (½ cup) F = 1
Kiwi Slices (½ cup)

Breakfast Fat Grams = 8

Snack:
Watermelon, cubed (1 cup)   Iced or Hot Herbal Tea

Snack Fat Grams = 0

Lunch:
Shrimp and Snow Pea, Spinach Salad with Lima Beans and Feta
  Jumbo Shrimp (3 oz.) F = 2   Snow Peas (1 cup)
  Baby Spinach (2 cups)   Lima Beans (¾ cup)
  Black Olives (8) F = 5   Feta Cheese (½ oz.) F = 4
Vinaigrette Salad Dressing, Low-fat (2 TB.) F = 5

Lunch Fat Grams = 16

Snack:
Real Ice Cream (½ cup) F = 9
Lemonade (sugar-free, sweetened with Stevia)

Snack Fat Grams = 9

Dinner:
Grilled Chicken Kabobs
  Mushrooms, Onion, Bell Pepper Chunks (1 cup)
  Chicken (3 oz.) F = 3
  Canola Oil (1 tsp.) F = 5
  Steamed Asparagus Tips (1 cup)
  Black Beans and Corn (½ cup) F = 1
Cantaloupe (1 cup)

Meal Fat Grams = 9

Snack:
Fresh Apple (1 small)

Snack Fat Grams = 0

Total Fat Grams for Friday = 42

Saturday:

Breakfast:
Poached Eggs (2) F = 10
Zucchini/Tomato Stir-fry
  Zucchini/Tomato, cooked (1 cup)   Olive Oil (1 tsp.) F = 5
Whole-grain Pumpernickel Bread (1 oz. Slice) F = 1
Honeydew Melon Cubes (1 cup)

Breakfast Fat Grams = 16

Snack:
Dates (3)   Herbal Tea

Snack Fat Grams = 0

Lunch:
Turkey and Pasta Salad with Blue Cheese
  Turkey Breast (3 oz.) F = 3   Blue Cheese (½ oz.) F = 4
  Baby Greens (2 cups) with Sliced Onions and Chopped Basil
  Spiral Whole-wheat Pasta, cooked al dente (⅓ cup) F = 1
  Creamy Italian Dressing (1 TB.) F = 5
Lentil Soup
  Lentils, cooked (½ cup)   Onions/Carrots, chopped

Lunch Fat Grams = 13

Snack:
Dried Peaches (4 halves)
Herbal Tea

Snack Fat Grams = 0

Dinner:
Poached Salmon with Rosemary (3 oz.) F = 9
Steamed Broccoli Spears Parmesan
  Broccoli (1 cup)   Parmesan Cheese (1 TB.) F = 1
Baked Yams (½ cup)
Yogurt, Plain Non-fat (6 oz.)
Butter (½ tsp.) F = 3

Dinner Fat Grams = 13

Snack:
Fresh Pear (1 small)   Herbal Tea

Snack Fat Grams = 0

Total Fat Grams for Saturday = 42

Sunday:

Breakfast:
Steel-cut Oats and Bran with Raisins and Nuts
  Oats (¼ cup dry, ½ cup cooked)
  Unprocessed Bran (¼ cup dry, ½ cup cooked)
  Raisins (2 TB.)
  Walnuts (6 halves) F = 8
Cottage Cheese and Pineapple
  2 percent Cottage Cheese (¾ cup) F = 3   Pineapple, unsweetened (½ cup)

Breakfast Fat Grams = 11

Snack:
Dried Apricots   Apricots (8, halves)

Snack Fat Grams = 0

Lunch:
Lean Roast Beef (3 oz.) F = 9 Au Jus
Steamed Cabbage Confetti (2 cups)
  Tomatoes, chopped (½ cup)
  Red Peppers, cut lengthways (½ cup)
  Cabbage, Shredded (1 cup)
Baked Butternut Squash with Cinnamon (1 cup)
Whipped Peaches and Cream
  Peaches, no sugar, canned (½ cup)   Cream (1 TB.) F = 5

Lunch Fat Grams = 14

Snack:
Fresh Mango Slices (½ cup)   Herbal Tea

Snack Fat Grams = 0

Dinner:
Baked Chicken Breast (3 oz.) F = 3
Herb Brussels Sprouts (1 cup)
New Red Potatoes with Skin (½ cup)
  Butter (1 tsp.) F = 5
Arugula and Baby Greens with Apple Slices
  Greens (2 cups)   Apple Slices (½ cup)
Caesar Salad Dressing (2 TB.) F = 9
Red Wine Vinegar (as desired)

Meal Fat Grams = 17

Snack:
Yogurt, Plain Non-fat (½ cup)
Strawberries (⅔ cup)

Snack Fat Grams = 0

Total Fat Grams for Sunday = 42

The Least You Need to Know

◆ The American Heart Association recommends that a person eat 30 percent or fewer of their calories from fat per day.

◆ The menus in this chapter are based on eating 1,500 calories a day and about 25% fat calories.

◆ Be sure to eat at least 20 percent dietary fat to stay healthy and facilitate weight loss.

Chapter 17

Weight-Loss Solutions for Children and Teens

In This Chapter

- ◆ Knowing whether your child is overweight
- ◆ Health problems that lead to weight gain
- ◆ Setting up family lifestyle guidelines
- ◆ Signs of eating disorders

Overweight children suffer. They suffer because they deal with ridicule and rejection from their peers. Often they can't participate in athletic activities or other school- and community-sponsored events. In a sense, they're victims of our fast-food, high-calorie, supersized world of eating and our inactive and leisurely lifestyle.

Even more important, overweight children are at risk for chronic diseases later in life, and, increasingly, even while they are still young. Incidences of heart disease, high blood pressure, and type 2 diabetes, once unheard of in the young, have dramatically increased as young people become more overweight and obese. Other possible health effects of childhood obesity and being overweight are metabolic syndrome, elevated triglycerides, hormonal imbalances, and skin disorders.

Quite often, weight issues for children are a family affair. In this chapter, we discuss causes of childhood weight gain and solutions you can start using today to help your child or teen lose weight and regain their health, self-esteem, and well-being.

Is Your Child Overweight?

You might not be able to tell by looking. The BMI charts designed for adults don't work for children and teens. You'll need to use different techniques to determine whether your child needs to lose weight and how much. Here are some tools you can use singly or in combination.

- **The standard weight charts at the doctor's office.** If your child's weight is 120 percent or higher than normal for his or her age and height, he or she is considered obese. Use the following charts as a reference.

- **Body fat percentage.** Ask your health-care practitioner or at the fitness center whether they can measure your child's body fat percentage. This is an easy way to determine whether your child is overweight or obese.

  Boys: Obese if body fat is 25 percent or higher. Overweight if body fat is between 21–25 percent. Healthy range is between 9–15 percent.

  Girls: Obese if body fat is 32 percent or higher. Overweight if body fat is between 22–31 percent. Healthy range is between 14–21 percent.

- **Modified BMI Chart.** The Centers for Disease Control and Prevention uses a modified BMI chart that accounts for age and normal growth rates—one chart for boys and one for girls. But the BMI charts don't give accurate information for persons with high muscle mass, such as athletes, so be careful in using this tool. Use the following charts.

You can use all or any of the tools listed here. We recommend that you use body fat percentage as a gauge for your child and for yourself. That way, you'll avoid the drudgery and fear of stepping on the scales. Plus, you'll have a more accurate measurement.

Boys: 2 to 20 years

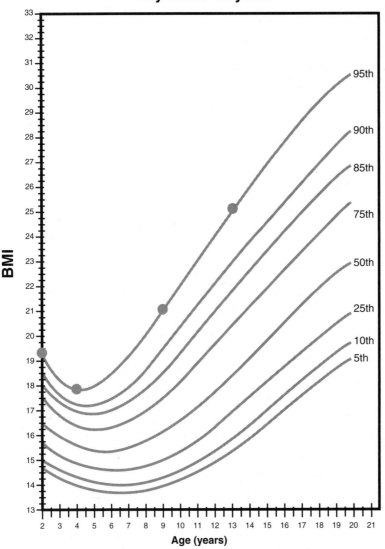

BMI chart for boys.

BMI chart for girls.

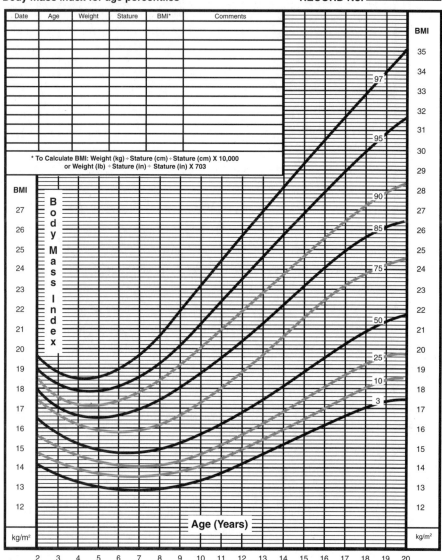

Set Goals

Establish body fat percentage goals for your child at 3, 6, and 9 months from now, and a year into the future. Measure the body fat only at these intervals. More frequent measuring won't accurately reflect the changes, as they happen slowly. An excellent goal would be to reduce body fat by one to two percentage points every three months. In other words, if your daughter now has a body fat percentage of 30 percent, at the end of one year, a body fat percentage of somewhere around 24–25 percent would represent great success. Then keep going until you've reached your ideal. Hurrying isn't important; health is.

Celebrate each percentage point lowered with a special treat—one that doesn't involve food. Decide ahead of time with your child what the treat will be. It can be a trip to the amusement park, a new soccer ball, new clothes, an overnight slumber party, or any number of other fun rewards.

Weighty Warning

If you think your child is a little bit pudgy, don't panic. Don't pull out the diet books and clear out the refrigerator. Children grow in leaps and spurts. They can be a bit pudgy for a couple of months and then grow two or three inches within a half year. Then they'll be in the normal range of weight. Take a calmer and more scientific approach. Your emotions will benefit, and so will theirs.

Checking Out Health Factors

You're looking for solutions that will help your child. Your first impulse could be to restrict food and regulate eating. Don't do this at first. Your child could be overweight for other reasons that are related to health and his or her body.

Be sure that you understand the full picture of your child's situation before you take any action. Otherwise, you can unknowingly contribute to your child developing a "fat mentality" for no reason.

Check out the following factors first when your child is overweight: allergies, celiac disease, drugs (prescription and illegal), type 2 diabetes, and genetics. Each will be described in the sections that follow.

Allergies

Food allergies as well as food sensitivities can cause weight gain. Yes, it's possible to have no other symptoms. You can't count on seeing runny noses or sneezes with some food sensitivities. Instead, a person's body perceives the food as a poison and limits digestion of nutrients, thus causing the body to store fat.

The most common foods that cause allergies and sensitivities are wheat, dairy, and soy. Second to those are aspartame and other artificial sweeteners. An allergic reaction to sugar is possible, too.

One easy way to determine whether your child is sensitive to a food is to use an elimination diet. For one week, have your child not eat any wheat. If they lose weight in that week, wheat could be the problem. Do the same the next week for dairy, and then for soy and then sugar.

If you find a food culprit, eliminate it from his or her diet. Of course, that's easier said than done. But limiting allergenic foods is definitely easier than spending many futile years dieting with no long-term results.

You can find excellent books and cookbooks on living a wheat-free, dairy-free, or soy-free life.

Another choice is to take your child to an allergist for testing to determine if your child has allergies or food sensitivities and for food and eating recommendations.

Celiac Disease

Celiac disease is a chronic digestive disorder caused by an inherited intolerance to gluten. Symptoms can be irritable bowel syndrome, diarrhea, and weight gain or loss.

As many as 1 out of 500 people in the United States have celiac disease. A cure for the condition doesn't exist, but it can be solved by eliminating gluten-containing foods from the diet. The foods that contain gluten are wheat, oats, seminola, spelt, rye, barley, triticale, and kamut.

If you suspect that your child can't tolerate gluten, have him or her tested by an allergist to confirm or dispel your suspicions. The allergist can give you further resources for helping your child make healthy and allergy-free food choices.

Drugs—Prescription and Illegal

Some prescription medications can cause weight gain and also stall or thwart weight loss. Steroid-based medications such as prednisone and those used in asthma inhalers are the worst. So are some anti-seizure medications. If your child is on one of these, ask the doctor whether other medications available won't cause weight gain.

Abuse of some prescription medications can cause weight gain. These are usually pain killers or anti-anxiety drugs.

Illegal drugs are never a fun topic, but use of recreational drugs can cause weight gain or loss. The most notable is marijuana, but also others that soothe and relax. Having a post-marijuana attack of the "munchies" is an obvious way to gain weight.

If you suspect your child is using drugs recreationally, seek counseling to learn how to effectively talk with your child. Cessation of the drug use will be the big gain, but your child may be able to lose some excess weight, too.

Type 2 Diabetes

Type 2 diabetes was formerly called "adult-onset diabetes." That was true until more and more younger people were being diagnosed with it. To accommodate the children who had this form of diabetes, it was renamed.

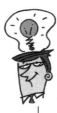

Thinspiration

As you help clear up your child's health conditions, you also help your child to release stored excess body fat and to live a well-balanced life.

If your child has Type 2 diabetes, it'll be harder for them to lose weight. The same is true if they have metabolic syndrome, which is the precursor to Type 2 diabetes. Elevated triglyceride levels, weight gain, elevated fasting blood sugar levels, and high blood pressure characterize metabolic syndrome. If you suspect your overweight child could have metabolic syndrome, consult with a doctor. You, your child, and your doctor working together can prevent it turning into full-blown diabetes.

When a person is on medication for Type 2 diabetes, it's harder to lose weight. This is true for insulin as well as oral medications. Your child and you need to meet with a CDE—certified diabetes educator—or a Registered Dietitian to learn how to eat to stabilize blood sugar levels and lose weight.

Genetics

Being overweight or having a tendency to store excess body fat can be genetic. But not always. The medical conditions of celiac disease and diabetes have genetic roots.

If your children are also your biological children, you're already prepared for this possibility. But if your child is adopted, you often have no way to know. If you have suspicions that your child might be genetically disposed to health conditions that cause weight gain, don't wait. Consult with a doctor or specialist, get the necessary testing done, and find out the answers. Then you have the ability to assist your child.

Parents as the Problem

Don't be a parent who panics if a child is overweight. The situation can be solved. But not if you get in the way. Yes, this is tough talk, but we've seen it too often. For example:

♦ A parent who compulsively puts her 9-year old daughter on a highly restrictive diet when she's only 10 pounds above normal weight. We suspect the mother fears social pressure more than the daughter.

♦ A parent who suggests to her preteen that they embark on a formal diet program together, and attend meetings, and so on. Let her be a child. Too much pressure, too-high expectations. And the mother is in a sense making the daughter responsible for the mother's success at losing weight.

♦ A parent who sends her 16-year-old daughter to a weight-loss coach and then refuses to let the daughter eat as recommended. This is craziness.

♦ A parent who refuses to acknowledge that the child is overweight and who does nothing.

All of these are bad examples and usually end up making matters worse. To help you maneuver your way through the steps to helping your child, we've put together suggestions for what to do first, then next, and so on to create a positive and healthy solution.

The Eating Environment

Overweight children come from all kinds of families: large families, busy families, single-parent families, low-income families, and high-income families. So do children who are at their ideal size for their age and height. There's no set formula.

However, you can create an environment that supports a healthy lifestyle for your child to live at his or her ideal size. Here are some suggestions:

Thinspiration

Try this breakfast experiment to break the cereal-on-the-run habit. Without asking anyone, fix a nice bowl of scrambled eggs and a plate of apples or oranges cut into pieces. Put them on the table and watch how readily your children gobble up this "new" breakfast. Cooking time: only 5–10 minutes.

- ◆ Serve or provide a good breakfast with animal protein and fruit or vegetables. Most children like scrambled eggs, ham, or other simple-to-prepare breakfast proteins. Leftovers will work, too.

- ◆ To control portion size, put food on plates at the stove and don't serve family style. Don't put bowls of food on the table and let everyone serve themselves.

- ◆ Discourage going back for seconds.

- ◆ Provide 5–10 servings of vegetables or fruits daily.

- ◆ Don't stock up on processed foods, whether frozen or packaged.

- ◆ Don't serve diet sodas and diet foods. Avoid sodas altogether. Just don't buy them or serve them infrequently.

- ◆ Serve healthy snack foods and eliminate snacks such as potato chips, popcorn, corn ships, and pretzels from the pantry. Avoid buying the sweet-tasting snacks such as cookies, muffins, breads, cakes, and candy except on special occasions.

- ◆ Eat dinner together as a family as often as you can.

- ◆ Model good and healthy eating behavior as explained in other sections of this book.

- ◆ Teach your child how to eat based on his or her physical food needs, such as eating 0–5.

- Make regular exercise a part of family life. Go swimming, hiking, or biking. Play tennis, racquetball, basketball, or other sports together and make it fun.

- Emphasize body fat percentage over weight.

- Lobby your school board to remove sodas, candy bars, and salty snack foods from vending machines. Suggest they replace them with bottled water and fresh fruit.

An unexpected positive consequence of helping an overweight child develop healthier habits is that it will improve the health and well-being of everyone in your family.

Lifestyle Factors

Before we give you this list, we want you to realize up front that making some of these changes could be tough to do. In fact, you might balk at these suggestions because, if you implement them, you'll need to make personal changes, too. But the bottom line is that making the lifestyle changes will help your child lose weight and keep it off. So here goes.

- Have set times for family eating and snacking. Turn off the TV when you eat meals. And no snacking when watching TV or working on the computer.

- Have a set time for "lights out" at bedtime. As best you can, ensure that your child sleeps 7–9 hours a night. Lack of adequate sleep often triggers weight gain.

Weighty Warning

On average, a child aged 8 to 18 is exposed to 8 hours and 33 minutes of media content every day. This comes mostly from television and radio. It translates into a whole lot of sitting or lying around. And a whole lot of inactivity. No wonder the ranks of overweight children have grown so much.

- Require that your child be involved in some form of extracurricular learning activity—things like chess club, art classes, acting, piano, or many other choices.

- Be sure that your child does some form of exercise or athletics daily. This means that you might need to shoot hoops with him or her after school and do recreational exercise alongside them, which will be good for everyone concerned.

- Don't center fun times, recreation, and family life around food and eating.

◆ Limit television viewing to one hour on school nights and two to three hours a day on the weekends.

◆ Remove the television set from your child's bedroom if you think it's a factor in your child being overweight. Ditto the computer if it interferes with sleep and interest in outside activities.

◆ Limit video games if you find your child is spending too much time immersed in playing, or you sense that he or she is addicted or compulsive about them.

◆ Make sure that your child gets outside for sunshine every day. We all need the great outdoors.

With these changes in place, you'll be setting up a supportive environment for your child to lose weight and to develop a healthy lifestyle throughout his or her life.

Thinspiration

One family with two school-age sons limits playing video games to 15 minutes at a time. Their sons earn the right to play video games by doing household chores. Perhaps you can set up a similar system in your house.

Supplements for Overweight Children

Your children need vitamins, minerals, and antioxidants, just as you do. Supply them with a high-quality children's formula, and when they reach their teens, give them an adult formula. This will meet most of their needs.

Make certain that your children eat enough fiber and roughage to ensure that they have regular bowel movements. (Just don't tell them why, or you'll get an "Oh, mom, that's gross!" reaction!) You can, if necessary, supplement their fiber intake with a plain psyllium or a psyllium-based product, but make sure that it doesn't contain artificial sweeteners such as aspartame or Splenda.

Taking dietary supplements ensures that your child receives all the necessary nutrients he or she needs to build and maintain a healthy body. But supplements alone don't offer a magic bullet for weight loss. Think of them as support for weight loss and overall health while supplementing a healthy diet.

Avoid giving your child supplements specifically formulated for weight loss. No research has been conducted on the safety of these for children. Some of the ingredients might actually interfere with normal growth processes.

One very important "supplement" for weight loss is sunshine. The body needs at least 15 minutes of sunshine a day for the hormones to function properly. And that's important for people of all ages. So join your child outside to catch some rays.

Eating Disorders

Eating disorders usually start in adolescence. Their roots are psychological. The results can be devastating. They can ruin a person's quality of life and, in extreme cases, can lead to serious illness and death.

As a parent, you want to know the warning signs. Eating disorders affect both men and women, boys and girls. When the problems are caught early, children with eating disorders have an overwhelmingly good chance of correcting their eating behaviors and regaining their mental, emotional, and physical health.

Here are the warning signals:

◆ Overly high concern with body image. You'll be walking a fine line here, because adolescence is the time of acute body awareness and comparison with others. A high concern is normal. An overly high concern could lead to problems.

◆ Constantly telling everyone around them that they're fat. Some of this is normal, but too much is out of bounds.

◆ Overeating but not gaining weight. This could be the result of *bulimia*, which involves bingeing and purging (self-induced vomiting). Warning signs of bulimia include (1) making excuses to go to the bathroom right after meals; (2) odd smells emanating from the bathroom after meals, often covered up with room sprays and fresheners; and (3) use of laxatives or diuretics.

◆ Unexplained weight loss. This could be a sign of *anorexia*. The warning signs are (1) highly regimented eating patterns or not eating with family and friends; (2) thinking they're fat no matter how small they get; (3) denying feeling hungry; and (4) exercising excessively. Anorexics often become socially withdrawn.

◆ Eating large amounts of food and feeling guilty or acting secretive about it. This could be a sign of a binge-eating disorder.

If you suspect a problem, first do your research. Read about the problem, search the Internet, and consult with an expert. Solving the problem is beyond the ability of your family and friends. You need professional help. So does your child. Get it.

> **Lean Lingo**
>
> **Bulimia** is an eating disorder characterized by overeating and purging, or throwing up. It's harmful to a person's health. It's a serious psychological problem, so consult with a professional who specializes in eating disorders if you suspect your son or daughter could be bulimic. **Anorexia** is a psychological disease in which a person starves themselves seemingly to attain a very slim body. It's very serious and can lead to death. If you suspect that your son or daughter is anorexic, consult with a professional who specializes in eating disorders.

The Least You Need To Know

- Check for health-related weight-gain issues before starting your child on a weight-loss program.

- Set up family rules to discourage inactivity and reinforce exercise and outside activities.

- Model good eating behaviors, such as eating 0-5, eating nutrient-dense foods, and getting regular exercise.

- Be on the alert for warning signs of eating disorders.

Part 5

Exercise Is Your Friend

Exercise is one of the most inexpensive yet luxurious of life's pleasures. It helps you lose weight and is a significant factor in keeping your weight off. It lifts your moods and makes you feel good all over. So what's not to like about exercise? How about that it takes time and energy and feels like work, plus you are "supposed" to do it? This part of the book shows you how to do exercises that count the most toward getting in shape and how to enjoy every sweaty moment.

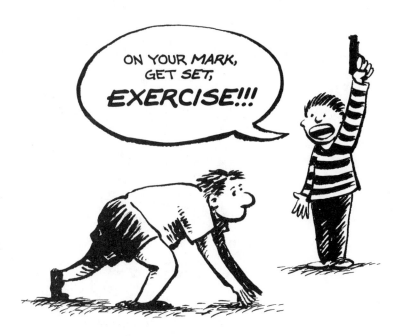

Chapter

18

Your Body Craves Exercise

In This Chapter

- ◆ Overcoming sedentary inertia
- ◆ Maintaining your ideal size
- ◆ Working at working out

Do you know what modern man is really good at? Sitting. We've really mastered the art of sitting. After all, it's a lot more comfortable to watch television sitting down, and watching television is our national pastime! And that's only part of our regular sitting routine. There's also driving to work, working at a desk, and sitting down for meals. In fact, most golfers even sit in little carts from one hole to the next.

What was once a necessary part of our ancestors' survival—movement—is pretty much optional today. Of course, we have a price to pay for becoming a sedentary nation. We're also getting flabbier. Our muscles maintain their shape from use. The less we use them—and it doesn't take a lot of muscle power to sit—the less shapely our muscles become. It's that simple.

But you already know this, right? So why don't you use your muscles more? For a thousand reasons, we're sure. Everyone can come up with oodles of reasons *not* to exercise. In this chapter, we ask you to take a fresh look at exercise, put aside your well-entrenched prejudices, and commit to a plan to exercise regularly and happily for the rest of your life.

Overcoming Exercise Inertia

Amidst the busy life you live, sometimes exercising is the last thing you want to do. You're tired. Your to-do list is packed with a dozen other things to take care of. Just the thought of exercising makes you exhausted! We know the feeling, too. Some days we have to force ourselves to exercise, but we do it. We do it because we know what happens when we don't, but mostly we enjoy it!

Inertia Has a Price Tag

Overcoming exercise *inertia* is a critical step toward reaching your ideal body size. When we don't exercise, all kinds of unpleasant side effects occur. Our legs get flabby; our waists become bigger; and our upper arms jiggle like Jell-O. We struggle to find enough energy to get through the day. We seem to become more anxious and perhaps a bit depressed—feelings that often lead us right to the kitchen searching for something to eat.

Lean Lingo

In physics, the law of **inertia** states that a body in motion tends to stay in motion and a body at rest tends to stay at rest. The same is true for a person and movement. Thus, according to this law, a person who exercises tends to do more activity overall, and a person who is sedentary tends to stay among the couch potatoes.

From a health point of view, exercise inertia can be fatal. You reduce your risk of virtually every chronic disease—diabetes, cancer, high blood pressure, heart disease, autoimmune disorders and more—with regular vigorous exercise. As an added benefit, exercise improves your health if you have one of those disorders.

When we don't exercise regularly, we feel like, well, like slugs. And that doesn't feel good. We like ourselves less. Even our postures sag.

This is probably not the image you want for yourself. Right? Your ideal self-image is instead loaded with positive attributes—great posture, bright eyes, firm upper arms, and a flat tummy. Well, the road that takes you toward your ideal body size involves exercise along the way. In other words, plan to exercise regularly to get what you want.

Positive Self-Talk About Exercise

Many people tell themselves that they hate to exercise. This kind of negative internal self-talk is sure to make matters worse. As we've suggested throughout this book, your mind is your most powerful tool to help you reach your ideal size, so use it wisely when it comes to exercise. Don't talk about or even think about exercise in negative terms. Instead, tell yourself the following:

> "I love to exercise."
> "It feels good to exercise."
> "I would rather exercise than sit around at night."
> "I love to take walks during lunch."
> "I love to go out dancing."
> "I enjoy going to the gym and working out."
> "I enjoy my aerobics classes."
> "I like to play tennis, golf, racquetball, and so on."
> "I enjoy my home exercise program."
> "I smile after a good workout."

The more you can program yourself to enjoy exercise, the easier for you to overcome exercise inertia.

Dealing with Your Barriers

Of course, it's not just negative thoughts that keep you from exercising. You have *real* reasons not to exercise, right? Let's think about them and see whether you can get past them.

No Time!

I don't have time to exercise. Of course you don't. We've found that basically no one has time to exercise. People don't become regular exercisers because they were bored and didn't have anything else to do. Exercise can seem so frivolous when so many other "important" things must get done.

Broaden your viewpoint. Without enough regular exercise, you're more likely to lack the energy and stamina to tackle all your chores, to feel good at the end of the day instead of exhausted, and to reach your ideal size.

There is no way around your need to exercise. You can't hire someone to do it for you. You can't have it done to you passively while you rest. You can't do just a little and expect huge results. You can't speed it up and do it in less time. Exercise takes as much time as it takes. Even money can't buy you exercise.

If you're really struggling to find time to exercise, get creative. When Helen was a mom with a six-month-old, she would head to the park with her baby in the stroller. There she would run circles on a wide path around the stroller so she could get in her running. Undoubtedly she might have gotten a few curious stares from onlookers, but it worked.

Today, most health clubs offer childcare, so you can still get in a workout. Or you could develop a home program if you've got small children. Exercise during naptime, when they're in the playpen, or while they play at your feet. You'll find it worthwhile even if it's not your ideal. And don't forget your spouse! Ask him or her to baby-sit while you work up a sweat and enjoy exercising for a half hour.

Put it on your schedule. Don't rely on "when you feel like it" exercising. Schedule exercise into your daily agenda and make sure that you block off at least 45 minutes three times a week—or more. Plan to schedule exercise for the rest of your life. Intermittent bursts of exercise are okay, but they don't add up to much over your lifetime. You never outgrow your need for exercise.

Thinspiration

There really aren't shortcuts to exercise. Perhaps that's the real beauty of it. Could it be that your exercise time is time just for you? Time to de-stress, to decompress, to be alone with your thoughts? Time to enjoy some of the sensuous pleasures of your body's movement and sweat?

What About My Hair!

I hate what exercising does to my hair! Unless you're bald or you shave your head, there's a good chance that working up a sweat will mess up your hair. Yuck! Wouldn't it be great if you could exercise hard without wrecking your hairstyle or needing to shower afterward?

This problem can only be tackled through practical measures and a good attitude. The best attitude to adopt is that *not* exercising wrecks a heck of a lot more than exercising ever can. Not exercising wrecks your weight-loss progress, lowers your metabolic rate, and erodes your health. So what's a hairstyle and more antiperspirant when we're talking about your ideal size and health?

Carefully choose the type of exercise and the timing of your exercise to handle your showering and hair concerns. Many of us prefer to exercise in the morning before work. Some prefer after work. Noontime aerobics classes are a bit harder for handling personal hygiene, but you can solve the problem if you're motivated enough. How about an easier-to-manage hairstyle?

Embarrassed at the Health Club

Health clubs intimidate me. Do you find yourself comparing other bodies to yours? Do you believe that others at the gym are looking at your body critically, especially if you're not yet at your ideal size? Or even if you are? We have clients who are embarrassed to be seen riding their bicycles in public. They feel that every passerby is commenting on the size of their thighs. How do you overcome this?

We certainly don't recommend hiding out because you aren't in the shape or at the size you want to be. You can start your exercise program at home. Terrific exercise videos are available, and home exercise equipment is a great investment … if you use them (check out Appendix B for more information). Chapter 21 will show you how to set up an at-home exercise plan. You can also join a health club or go to the local rec center and exercise. Just be sure to not compare your body to others; rather, use the time as your personal time for you. Luxuriate in the pleasure of moving your body, the sweat, and the heavy breathing.

By all means, do as much exercise out of doors as you want. If a passerby has thoughts about your body, well, only you know how mistaken and petty that person is. He or she is passively riding in a car; you, on the other hand, are getting fresh air, sunshine, and terrific body movement.

Exercise Is Hard and It Hurts

Whenever I start exercising again, my body is so sore. Yes, we don't disagree. At first, you can be stiff and sore after an especially energetic workout. It can be hard to catch your breath, your lungs can feel as though they can't get enough oxygen, you can feel really out of shape. In this situation, you only have two choices—stay out of shape or get in shape.

The only way out is to go through it. You can go more slowly and let your body build stamina and muscle strength without so much huffing and puffing, wheezing, and stiffness.

Last year, Lucy moved to a small city within 15 minutes of the mountains and great hiking trails. "I thought I was in great shape until I started hiking. Oh my gosh, after a half hour my legs were mush, and they wobbled. My heart pounded. I got woozy but didn't want anyone, namely my husband, to know. After several hikes, he started watching me more carefully. When my legs started trembling as I climbed, he made me stop and take my pulse rate. [Do this by counting the pulse on your wrist or neck for 6 seconds and multiply by 10.] If my heart rate was too high, say over 140, he had us turn around and head down the mountain. I didn't like this because I wanted to reach the top. However, by not pushing myself to the top early on, over the summer, I developed the stamina to go farther and farther every hike. Now those same hikes feel like a cakewalk."

Muscle soreness and stiffness on the days after exercise is caused by a build-up of lactic acid in your muscles. To feel better, drink lots of water, stretch your sore muscles, and take hot Epsom salt baths. You can tell by now that we recommend baths for almost any condition. The luxury of massages is great, too.

The Value of You

Regular exercise isn't just about the many benefits; it is about the value of you. What is your intrinsic value to yourself, your family, and the world? As you value yourself and your contributions, you understand that taking care of yourself is essential to giving to others. Just a note here: if you are a caretaker or are in a care-giving career, it is very important that you take care of you. Many overweight people are primary caregivers and forget to also care for themselves.

Demonstrate your own self-esteem and self-worth by taking good care of yourself through exercise.

Boost Your Metabolism

Exercise boosts your metabolic rate. As you exercise, you increase your muscle mass, leading you to sport a higher metabolic rate. This means you burn through your food faster. Thus, you actually need to eat more food to stay at your ideal size.

For example, let's compare two women. Both are the same age and weight. The first woman works out by doing strength training three times a week. The other doesn't do any form of strength training. The first woman needs to eat more calories to stay at her ideal size than the other one—simply because she has more muscle and less fat on her body.

This is why. A pound of fat requires only three calories per pound for maintenance. A pound of muscle requires 35 to 50 calories per pound. It's highly beneficial to your weight loss to have a low body fat percentage and high muscle mass.

As we counsel our weight-loss clients, it's amazing how some of them need such little amounts of food while others need lots more. The ratio of body fat to muscle makes a big difference in how much food it takes to maintain your ideal size. A woman with a high body fat percentage, say at 40 percent, can eat such small amounts of food and still gain weight, while a woman with 20 percent body fat can eat way more food and stay at her ideal size. It doesn't seem fair.

Get your body fat down through strength training and use the "passive" activity of your higher metabolism to stay at your ideal size.

Maintain Your Ideal Size

We question whether a person can really lose weight through exercise alone. We've never seen this happen. We suppose that if a person went from being totally sedentary to running in marathons then he or she would lose weight. But a person could gain weight from exercise. Since muscle weighs more than fat, a person could do strength training and gain weight, yet fit into his or her clothes better. In other words, the person could be a smaller size and yet weigh more. At that point, who cares? The person looks great.

But research shows over and over again that the people who maintain weight loss are the people who continue to exercise over their lifetimes. This is because of the boost in metabolism and because exercise lifts mood, soothes anxiety, and improves health. When you feel good about yourself, you tend to make healthier decisions about food, eating, and your life.

Shape Comes from Muscles

If you lost a lot of weight and didn't exercise as you were losing, you might get to your ideal size, but you could never get close to your desired shape.

Joan started at a size 22. Within a year and a half, she was wearing a size 8. This is terrific. She exercised by doing the five Tibetan exercises (see Chapter 20) every day, and she rode her exercise bike three times a week. She looked terrific as a size 8, and you couldn't tell that she had ever been overweight.

Thinspiration _____

Sandy is a perfect example of being at her ideal size all her life. But as a result of getting older and letting her exercise regimen fall by the wayside, she put on too many inches. As she says, "I am intelligent and teach others this concept—I live with a triathlete and marathoner for goodness sake! I feel better when I exercise, ... but if I get out of the habit because of an extended vacation or whatever, it might take me months to get back into a regular routine again.

"Exercise isn't my top priority—I'd rather do other things. I am my best at exercise when I do it first thing in the morning and go to work a little later rather than trying to fit it in after work. My early evenings are not consistent, and after supper I am surely not going to rev up my exercise motor! The motivation to exercise needs to come from within. Know that at first, exercise ... won't be fun—but it has to be done—then it does become fun. Use a wide variety of exercise techniques so you don't get into a rut."

But if she hadn't exercised—oh, dear. Joan would have had sagging, loose skin all over her body. Her muscles would have been flabby. At that point, no amount of exercise could have firmed up the sagging, loose skin. Her only alternative would have been plastic surgery and lots of it.

Don't let this happen to you. If you exercise as you lose weight, your skin firms up and tones as you lose each ounce and pound. It shrink-wraps to fit your muscles. But if you don't strengthen, stretch, and do cardio, the damage can be irreparable. We want you to look good in your clothes and on the beach. If you think you may need some nips and tucks after weight loss, make sure to maintain your weight loss for at least nine months before you opt for surgery. Yes, we have friends who had the work done too soon and then gained the weight back. It's not a pretty picture.

Goodbye, Blues

Aerobic exercise produces wonderful brain chemicals called endorphins. To get them in circulation, you need to break a sweat and do at least 20 minutes of aerobics or cardio exercise with an elevated heart rate. Less just isn't enough.

The flood of endorphins has been called the runner's high. Endorphins make you feel good. They lift your moods, even for hours later.

If you experience late-afternoon blues, if you battle anxiety and depression, get your endorphin lift daily or at least three times a week. If you are an emotional eater, break the pattern by doing regular cardio workouts.

Our favorite story about the endorphin lift is about a woman who was so depressed she wanted to commit suicide. But she didn't want her family to suffer because of this, so she devised a plan to kill herself. She would go out running so hard and so long that she would die. Well, she didn't die the first day, so she set out the second day, and the third, and the fourth. Soon she felt so good that she no longer wanted to die; in fact, she wanted to live. She cured her own deep depression through using those endorphins.

We find it easier to do the cardio when we enjoy the day-to-day benefits of soothed anxiety and happier moods. This activity also forestalls lots of stress eating. Other activities that can soothe stress eating before it starts are found in Chapter 8.

> **Thinspiration**
>
> The road to reaching your ideal body size can't be driven to in the comfort of a Cadillac or SUV! Be prepared to walk, run, and skip—in other words, to exercise—along the way.

Exercise Your Mental Function

Recent studies show that people who exercise think better. They score better on tests. They exhibit more creativity than when they don't exercise. Yes, exercise improves brain functioning.

Do you want your children to get better grades? Go shoot hoops after school with them. Ride bikes with them or take them with you to the gym.

Do you want to be more creative or to perform better at work? Get your regular dose of exercise and do it for life. Exercise increases cerebral blood flow and stimulates nerve cell growth.

Energy

If you feel sluggish and low on energy, by now you know the solution: get out and move. In earlier chapters, you garnered eating suggestions to correct late-afternoon tiredness. Now add in exercise. You could look up at the clock and discover that you just sailed through the late afternoon, and it's already time to quit work or eat dinner.

You will have energy to keep up with the kids or your spouse. You will have energy to enjoy social activities in the evening and not collapse after dinner in front of the TV—but perhaps not at first. As Sandy says, "When I haven't exercised regularly, and I start up my exercise program again with aerobics in the mornings, I come in from my walk or finish my videotape and I am exhausted! I probably start back at the level where I left off a few months before. But that feeling of tiredness is worth it—it leads to regaining the energy I want!"

Overall, Your Health

The most significant activity for enjoying good health throughout your life is exercise. Nothing else counts as much. Food choices and supplements are important, but overall, nothing beats exercise for keeping you healthy.

Exercise helps you maintain weight loss, strengthens bones, eases hormonal difficulties, strengthens your heart, keeps blood pressure in a healthy range, and keeps your digestion and elimination functioning well. It even helps prevent certain forms of cancer.

What's not to like about exercise? Most likely, the fact that you have to do it. Make it a priority. Yes, we all have those days when we just don't want to do it. Taking a day off is fine. Taking two days off is risky. It is too easy to just stop entirely.

Do whatever it takes to exercise. Do it with a friend, schedule it into your daily agenda, do it with a trainer or your spouse or children. Do it, and the rewards will speak loudly.

Remember to get in motion. That is the best way to stay in motion.

The Least You Need to Know

- Exercise is essential for long-term weight maintenance.
- The inconveniences of exercise are insignificant compared to the enormous benefits.
- Exercise gives you the shape you want as you get to your ideal size, but it alone doesn't make you lose weight.
- Increasing muscle mass through strength training lowers your body fat content and boosts metabolism.
- The absolute best activity you can do for your overall health and for weight maintenance is to exercise regularly.

Chapter 19

The Essence of Exercise

In This Chapter

- ◆ Making friends with exercise
- ◆ Easing into a good exercise routine
- ◆ Using proper form—it matters
- ◆ Gaining health benefits
- ◆ Lightening your stress load

The essence of exercise is doing what your body was designed to do—use your muscles. Using your muscles is primitive. It's refreshing. It makes you feel good. It keeps you healthy. And regular exercise is a significant factor in helping you keep excess weight off for life.

Yes, some thin people do not exercise regularly. Are you one of them? Probably not. Can you claim any benefits to your health and weight loss from *not* exercising? Of course not. Let exercise become as routine and important to you as brushing your teeth. You wouldn't think of not brushing your teeth. Make it so that you wouldn't think of not exercising every day or every other day. It's that important.

Exercise Is Your Friend

Exercise is my friend? No way! Okay, we'll grant that most friends don't make you sweat, but you should get on good terms with exercise if you want to lose weight and keep it off. It works!

Regular exercise, if it includes both strength and cardio training, will boost your metabolic rate and help you burn fat more quickly. Recent studies show that subjects who didn't exercise had a reduced capacity to burn stored fat, both during exercise and when at rest. With regular exercise, you even burn more fuel when you sleep than if you are sedentary.

You can lose weight without exercising, but it will be harder to do, and you won't feel as energized. We're not talking about becoming a marathoner or gym-aholic. We want you to develop an exercise program that fits you, your body, and your lifestyle.

Even low-intensity exercise, such as walking briskly three times a week, might be adequate to prevent the post–weight-loss decline in the rate of fat burning. However, it's best to do cardio and strength training plus flexibility work because the health and fat-loss benefits are even more enticing.

What Doesn't Count as Exercise

Some forms of recreation just aren't going to give you good results for fat burning, an increase in metabolism, and overall excellent health. Some people want to think these are exercise, but they simply don't count. Some are obvious: billiards, television, video games, bridge, poker, and miniature golf, to name a few. Also, don't expect exercise benefits from bowling, horseshoes, golfing with a cart, hitting balls at the driving range, or fishing.

None of these activities count as exercise, but they can be fun and certainly are recreational. Enjoy them if you're so inclined, but you'll also need to have a real exercise plan.

Thinspiration

Start affirming your commitment to exercise ... even as you read this chapter. Don't give in to the negative self-talk that produces innumerable excuses for why you didn't or can't exercise. A positive attitude has helped countless individuals who were couch potatoes become fit and thin for life. You can do it!

Starting to Exercise

The hardest part about starting a personal exercise program is often just that—starting. For many of us, it's pretty intimidating. We become more self-conscious of our bodies and fear that we'll somehow "fail" at exercising. Your body is designed for motion and exercise. You'll do fine. To help you get off on the right foot, so to speak, the next few sections cover some things to consider.

Start Slow to Win the Race

If you start out at a level that is too tough for you, you might experience lots of pain and virtually no gain. Be sure to honor the current state of your body and your fitness level before you dive in. If you're out of shape, build up your strength and stamina. Remember that you're into exercise for the long haul, in essence, for the rest of your life. You can afford the time it takes to get your body into shape. When a person goes too quickly, the ensuing bodily aches and pains can prevent further exercise … and destroy motivation. Don't let this happen to you!

Remember the race between the tortoise and the hare? The tortoise started slowly but eventually won the race. When it comes to exercising, start slowly and build up your "speed" over time. You don't need to compete with anyone!

> **Thinspiration**
>
> By tuning in to your body wisdom, you can learn how to exercise to suit your personal needs. Just as you have learned how to eat based on your body's signals, you can learn how to exercise by listening to your body's instinctive knowing.

Clothing to Sweat In

Wear clothing appropriate to the type of exercise you're doing. Go for comfort and practicality. Some forms of exercise require more fitted leotards and tights. Some are fine with loose-fitting T-shirts and gym shorts. Forget how you look in exercise clothes and go for practicality and comfort. You're going to look better day after day.

You don't need to think that you are supposed to compete with all the beautiful and buff bodies at the gym. You are there to take care of yourself, just as they are. Wear what works and what feels comfortable.

Remember the Sunscreen

Exercises done outdoors—biking, hiking, running, walking, and so on—are a double treat for many of us because we get the added benefits of sunshine and fresh air. But use sunscreen. Your skin isn't designed to be cooked, not even browned! Skin cancer is a serious problem these days, and it isn't selective. It will attack the skin of a buff athlete as quickly as anyone else.

Pain Isn't Required

Forget the famous exercise motto of "no pain, no gain." It's great for jocks, jockettes, and gym junkies. At the beginning, just do the exercises and avoid the pain. Right now, you are easing into a life-long exercise program.

Always listen to your body for when it is time to stop an exercise and when it is time to push harder. This will prevent overdoing it and also under-doing it. In some exercise classes, instructors keep yelling for you to "Push it!" or "Go harder!" Unless you like being provoked, either ignore the instructor, listen to your body, or find another class. It's absolutely not essential for you to overexert yourself to the point of being exhausted or sore.

Many elegant exercise choices available today produce terrific strength and tone with virtually no pain. We tell all in the next chapter.

Body of Knowledge
An exercise physiologist can suggest alternative methods for different exercises to compensate for any medical or bodily conditions you have.

Doctor's Checkup

It's always a good idea to check with your doctor before you begin an exercise program, especially if you have a particular health concern, such as a heart condition or a bad back. Doctors almost universally encourage regular exercise. If you plan to engage the services of a personal trainer, work out in a class, or exercise with a group, make sure that the group leader knows of any physical limitations you may have.

An Intelligent Exercise Approach

Some self-discipline and common sense will go a long way toward making exercise effective for you. Remember that this is your exercise program; you're not in a military boot camp. If you have a limited range of motion, only go as far as you're comfortable with each exercise. It's tempting to try to keep up or even compete in group classes, but you don't need to do this. Ask the instructor's advice when necessary.

At one time, Mimi engaged the services of a personal trainer who came to her home three times a week. Even though she has a weak rotator cuff in her right shoulder, the trainer kept demanding that she work the shoulder in a way that was painful. He ignored her discomfort. What an insensitive lout! Later, her doctor explained that some people of northern European descent (such as herself) naturally had this condition, and surgery wasn't a good solution. His suggestion: do as much exercise as possible and stop short of the pain.

Weighty Warning

Your exercise program should be pain-free. If any part of your body hurts, stop immediately. Push yourself enough to get a good workout, but not so far that you get injured. Injuries ruin your momentum and require time for recovery.

Fortunately, most knowledgeable personal trainers won't make the same mistake. Be sure to check credentials and references if you engage the services of a personal trainer. If you have an injury or a specific muscle weakness, ask the trainer to show you how to strengthen the area or how to get the same results without further injuring yourself.

Darlene was enticed into a very intense weight-training program through the startling before and after pictures in the newspaper. The program was advertised as only one hour a week required to attain the perfect body. But, oh boy, what an hour it proved to be! In class one evening, Darlene was doing sit-ups with more than 40 pounds of weights—buckshot sewed into bags—resting on her stomach and midriff. Hard? You bet! She popped a rib out of place! Yes, the ambulance came.

You don't need to go to extremes to get fit, nor should you ever hurt yourself. Take it easy and reach your goal like the tortoise rather than the hare.

Spot Reducing

Spot reducing works … at times. If you have a puffy tummy and want to streamline it, you can. Spot reducing doesn't necessarily mean losing weight at one specific part of your body. It means tightening up or elongating certain muscle groups. Spot reducing needs to be part of a complete whole-body exercise program.

Stacy was about 5'1" and wanted to trim her thighs. She got on the Stairmaster day after day,

Body of Knowledge

Spot reducing works when your body is ready for it. It's hard to tell what body areas require special attention until you get close to your ideal size. Many things will change about your body as you lose weight and exercise, so be patient, and don't focus on spot reducing.

trying to whip those thighs into shape. And her hard work did produce a new shape—bigger thighs!

Why? Because her body shape and musculature was such that she had short thighbones. As she stepped and stepped, her thighs got stronger and stronger, packing on more and more muscle. Rather than elongating the muscles, she was bulking them up. A better choice for her would have been exercises that elongated her thigh muscles, such as yoga, Pilates, and stretching.

Push Beyond Your Limits

Part of the "game" of exercise is to gradually and continually push your body's limits. If right now your limit is running a half-mile, eventually you will be able to double that. Don't think of this as a competition or even that more is better. Just know that in a couple months, you'll want to do more because your body will be ready to do more.

> **Thinspiration**
>
> Keep on keeping on. The more you get into the flow of regular exercise, the more you will love doing it. The health and weight-loss benefits begin the minute you start your program, and they grow as you continue your program. Be prepared to keep getting better, stronger, and more in control of your body and your weight.

> **Lean Lingo**
>
> Clickers and **pedometers** are small devices that attach to one's waistband or belt. They measure how many steps a person takes. A common goal is to take 10,000 steps a day, which is equivalent to walking about 4 to 5 miles.

Moving Beyond Mere Movement

Don't confuse exercise with movement. Movement is better than being sedentary, but isn't enough for burning fat and increasing muscle. Movement includes simple activities such as walking, climbing a few flights of stairs instead of taking the elevator, or parking at the far end of a parking lot and walking the extra steps to the grocery store. These kinds of activities are low intensity, however, and don't increase your pulse rate enough to release endorphins, nor to build muscle mass, nor to make a significant reduction in body fat.

Activities such as walking are sure better for you than sitting around. Often people measure movement with clickers or *pedometers*. These register how many steps you take—in other words, how much you're moving. Studies show that on average, 10,000 clicks or steps a day will reduce blood pressure and lower cholesterol. Moving your body will make you stronger and will burn calories. Wearing a pedometer is like having a personal trainer on your hip, counting your results and silently urging you to move more.

Unfortunately, low-intensity movement exercises don't produce the same fat-burning benefits as a higher-intensity workout. Plus, a high-intensity workout boosts your metabolism and keeps it high for a while after your workout. To get the best shape, tone, and cardio benefits from exercise, you'll need to do more than move, but what a great way to start. As you progress, increase the cardio intensity and add in strength training and flexibility exercises regularly to have a complete workout.

Do Them Correctly

You'll be amazed at the extra benefits you'll get when you perform exercises correctly. It really does make a difference, and you don't want to waste one moment doing an exercise incorrectly. Learn the correct posture for using everything from your stationary exercise bike to weight-lifting equipment.

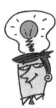

Thinspiration

Correct posture makes a big difference. If you're going to exercise at all, you may as well do it correctly.

Do you have any idea how many times we've seen people spend hours on a stair-stepping machine, slumped over the hand rails as if they need them to keep from keeling over. They might be doing some good, but they sure aren't getting the full benefit of the exercise. You can learn proper techniques from a trainer, a video, or a book. Get your form down right!

Exercise and Your Health

The single most significant factor in improving one's health is exercise. Research strongly indicates that exercise alone can improve your health, decrease the risk of serious illness, and reverse some of the degenerative effects of aging. Here's what exercise does for you:

- ◆ **Strengthens your heart.** The heart is a muscle, and it benefits from regular cardiovascular exercise, which means aerobics that will boost your heart rate. A stronger heart can avert arteriosclerosis and reduce high cholesterol and high blood pressure.

- ◆ **Increases lung capacity.** Exercise allows your lungs to increase their capacity to hold more oxygen. Exercise also lets your body use the oxygen it gets more efficiently, which increases your metabolism.

- **Increases bone density.** A woman who performs weight-bearing exercises regularly can increase her bone density and prevent the onset of osteoporosis. Studies show that even elderly women can benefit from weight-bearing exercise, such as lifting free weights or using the weight machines at the fitness center.

- **Improves insulin utilization.** Regular exercise lets your body reduce high levels of insulin, which reduces insulin resistance. High levels can lead to storing more fat, to metabolic syndrome, and ultimately, to Type 2 diabetes.

- **Helps prevent cancer.** Yes, you can reduce your risk of cancer by engaging in regular exercise.

- **Reduces the effects of aging.** Exercise improves muscle tone and counteracts the decrease in metabolic rate that comes with age.

- **Lessens depression and anxiety.** The release of endorphins that occurs after about 20 minutes of cardiovascular or aerobic exercise can lift one's mood for hours, perhaps even days. The endorphins soothe anxiety and reduce depression.

- **Increases mental acuity.** Studies indicate that people who exercise regularly have better mental alertness and prowess than those who don't.

Thinspiration

Instead of eating to tackle stress, work up a sweat. The endorphins released from 20 minutes of vigorous exercise can help you say good-bye forever to stress eating.

- **Helps balance hormones.** Hormones are responsible for energy, sex drive, moods, digestion, and many other bodily functions. Having balanced hormones can reduce the effects of aging and boost your energy.

The health benefits of regular exercise will let you enjoy living at your ideal size. We especially like that endorphin-stimulating exercise can reduce depression and lessen anxiety.

The Least You Need to Know

- People who maintain weight loss the best are those who exercise regularly.

- Start your exercise program slowly and work up gradually to optimum exercise levels.

- The health benefits of exercise are significant, contribute to overall well-being, and reduce the effects of aging.

- Regular exercise will help you reduce the anxiety that often brings on overeating.

Chapter 20

Variety Is the Spice of Exercise

In This Chapter

- ◆ The three basic types of exercise
- ◆ The great variety of exercise choices
- ◆ Wise exercise choices
- ◆ Exercise can be fun
- ◆ The fabulous five Tibetans

You should include three health-related fitness components in your exercise program: a cardio-respiratory component (aerobic/cardio), a muscle strength and endurance component (strength training), and a flexibility component (stretching).

Yes, you need to have all three activities in your exercise program (including warm-up and cool-down). Why? Because you deserve all the wonderful results. Here's the good news: many exercises encompass all three areas, and we'll show you which ones.

Aerobic/Cardio Exercise

Over the past 20 years the term "cardio" has gradually replaced the term "aerobic," but in this chapter we're going to use them interchangeably. The basic premise is simple: you need to exercise vigorously enough to speed up your heart rate and keep it up for at least 20 minutes. Why 20 minutes? Because it takes at least that long for your heart to work hard enough for you to experience cardiovascular and endorphin benefits.

That's right, get your heart rate up and keep it up for at least 20 minutes per session, ideally daily. Huff and puff a little. Break out in a sweat. Burn energy. Move fast. Vigorous aerobic exercise for 45 minutes every other day is a good alternative.

> **Thinspiration**
>
> The amount of recommended exercise can sound intimidating at first. Don't let it stop you. Start your exercise program slowly and work up to the recommended amount. No matter what shape you are in now, within a couple months, you'll be delighted with your progress. Stay with it.

Cardio builds your endurance, strengthens your heart, and increases your lung capacity. It releases endorphins, those wonderful mood-elevating brain chemicals. Exercise is one time when harnessing the power of drugs is fine because your body is making them. They're legal; they're free; and in fact, they're a natural high that your body is meant to enjoy.

You've got a lot of choices for the cardio/aerobic part of your workout. Choose one or more that you can do every day or every other day. They don't need to be fancy or elaborate. If you have a stationary bike, just schedule yourself to start peddling. Your simple goal is to elevate your heart rate for 20 minutes or more. At clubs and fitness centers, you can watch television. Listen to music on headphones, or read while you work up a sweat on the various cardio machines. However you do it, get your cardio exercise.

Here are target heart rates based on your age. Choose the age closest to yours. Try to keep your heart rate between the minimum and maximum for the duration of your cardio workout.

Age	Minimum	Moderate	Maximum
20	125	145	165
30	120	138	155
40	115	130	145
50	110	125	140
60	105	118	130
70	95	110	125
80	90	103	115

Measure your heart rate this way: Count your pulse by touching your fingers to the opposite wrist or to the pulse point in your neck. Count beats for 6 seconds. Multiply by 10 and that is your heart rate. If your heart rate stays close to the minimum target range for your age, increase your exercise session beyond 20 minutes or pick up the pace.

Here are some super choices for cardio/aerobic exercise:

◆ **Biking.** Bike either outdoors on a street bike or mountain bike or indoors on a stationary bike. It's terrific for low-stress, high-intensity aerobic fitness. Your only cost is the cost of your equipment—a stationary bike or one for the outdoors.

◆ **Classes.** A vast variety of aerobic fitness classes are available: step classes, aerobic dancing classes, spinning classes, power pump classes, and classes like Jazzercise. Fitness classes are widely available at health clubs, studios, and local recreation centers.

◆ **Cardio equipment.** These include treadmills, cross-country-skiing machines, elliptical trainers, stepping machines, and rowing machines. Most health and fitness facilities offer all of these and more. Find the ones you like the best and start moving. Many motels and hotels provide an exercise room with equipment, so you can exercise easily when you travel.

◆ **Cardio/aerobic videotapes.** Hundreds of good routines are available on video and DVD. Videos let you exercise at home without having to go out and can save you time. See Appendix B for sources of videos.

◆ **Swimming.** Swimming is great exercise, either indoors or outdoors, and indoor pools make swimming a year-round option. The expense involved is a health club or pool membership. Swimming also elongates muscles; we like that.

Thinspiration

Walking is excellent at the beginning of your exercise program. As you progress, however, we urge you to add in more strenuous exercise that gives you more cardio/aerobic benefits and that releases those uplifting endorphins. Walking alone won't give you that lift. That's why it's called the "runner's high," not the "walker's high!" However, if you speed walk while sustaining a moderately elevated heart rate as indicated above for 20 minutes or more, you could indeed, benefit from the runner's high by walking.

◆ **Walking.** Plain old walking can count as cardio/aerobic exercise if you can get your heart rate up to the moderate level or higher. But to do that, a casual stroll won't work. You've got to walk *fast*. We have friends who walk outdoors in good weather and who walk in shopping malls when it's raining or snowing. Some walkers enhance their workout by wearing shoes with weighted soles. These improve muscle tone in the lower body and increase the amount of physical energy expended. Sandy wears weighted shoes during work hours at the hospital. She finds them a great way to intensify her walking throughout the day. Plus she enjoys the lower-body firming from wearing them. (See Appendix B for more information on weighted shoes.) Avoid using ankle weights when you walk or climb stairs. They put too much stress on the ankle and knee joints and can cause harm.

◆ **Jogging, running, and race walking.** Purchase a good pair of shoes and go enjoy the outdoors. Unlike noisy gym classes, these activities give you an opportunity to take in beautiful scenery and off-street trails as you get fit and burn fat.

◆ **Rebounding using a mini trampoline or rebounder boots.** These give you a bouncing effect—kind of like bouncing on a pogo stick. Rebounding gets your endorphins flowing faster than many other forms of cardio/aerobic exercise, and it feels great. Some research shows that rebounding can be detoxifying for the body (great!) because it may stimulate the flow of lymph fluid. We like the rebounding boots for both jogging outside and doing aerobic dancing indoors. You can find more info on rebounding boots in Appendix B.

Rebounder boots are great for cardio exercise that energizes your endorphins.

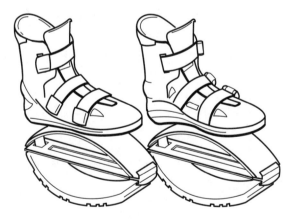

Strength Training—Get Strong

Strength training! But I don't want to look like Arnold Schwarzenegger! Good. Because that's not what we're talking about. Basic strength training is essential to increase your muscle tone, give your muscles shape and strength, and increase your metabolic rate. It helps alter your body composition from flabby fat to calorie-gobbling muscles and will make weight control much, much easier.

Strength training is also excellent for keeping your bones strong and avoiding osteoporosis in both men and women, for reducing your body fat percentage, and increasing your stamina.

Today, you have many excellent exercise choices for strength training. Once the only viable choice was using free weights or weight-training machines. They have stood the test of time. Today, however, you have other alternatives that work equally well. We know of several women who have reduced their body fat percentages by 10 points—say from 28 percent to 18 percent, or from 38 percent to 28 percent—just by doing core conditioning (also known as Pilates-type exercises) in one-hour sessions, two times a week, for six months.

Body of Knowledge

Strength training is more than essential—you need it to look and feel your best. The use of weights and resistance put greater than normal stress on your muscles, joints, and bones. (Just imagine lifting a dumbbell.) Under this strain, you create tiny, harmless tears in the muscle fibers. When you rest for a day or so between strength-training sessions, the muscles heal, resulting in stronger and more clearly defined muscles. As an added bonus, you'll have less body fat, too.

Strength training can turn upper arms from flabby into sexy. Ditto backs, thighs, and tummies. It improves posture. The key to building terrific muscles is to keep upping the intensity of your workout over time. Gradually increase the weight and the resistance as you get stronger. For example, when two- or three-pound weights get easy for your arm exercises, it's time to use five-pound weights.

Thinspiration

You can miss a week or two of strength training, but it will begin to show quickly in how your clothes fit … or don't. Thank goodness that when you restart your strength-training program, the results return quickly.

Here's a quick look at several forms of strength training. Find one or two that you enjoy and can do at least two sessions a week of one hour duration each. Don't do strength training every day. Rest at least one day between each session. Each of these choices offers different benefits, but when doing strength training, make sure to include exercises for your whole body. Work every muscle group. Also, be attentive to form and breathing, because proper technique makes a big difference in your overall results.

- **Free weights.** Barbells and dumbbells are great for developing your major muscles and may be used to create bulk. The number of repetitions and the speed of repetitions will affect the results you get. It's essential that you use free weights in the correct alignment; otherwise, your efforts will be wasted. Learn how before you embark on free-weights training. You can learn from an instructor, a book, or a video. You can use free weights at the gym and also set up a home program. Using free weights doesn't develop flexibility or elongate muscles, so be sure you add flexibility exercises to your program.

- **Weight-training machines.** These are available in most health clubs and fitness centers. The machines work major muscles and are easy to use because they help ensure proper alignment. You can also purchase these machines for your home. Keep in mind that these machines don't increase flexibility or lengthen muscles.

- **Core conditioning or Pilates.** These exercises can be done in a studio or class with an instructor or at home with videos or a book. They emphasize careful and precise movements to strengthen the body's core muscles in the abdomen area. All of the exercises, even for arms and legs, are done with a focus on using the core abdominal muscles for stability. Pilates programs work all the muscles: the major muscles and the smaller muscles. A big plus is that Pilates develops strength, elongated muscles, and flexibility. For many, it quickly improves posture. A side benefit: it's highly relaxing.

Body of Knowledge

A highly effective and efficient way to do strength training is what's known as Super Slow. Using this technique, you slow down your movements so that it takes two, three, or four times longer to do each repetition. Advocates say muscles get more of a workout because they're working constantly and don't get an easier ride because of the momentum of more rapid repetitions. The Super Slow approach works for almost all types of strength training.

◆ **Fitness ball.** These large balls, which range from 45 cm to 75 cm in diameter, promote strength and balance plus stretching. The exercises look simple, but the extra challenge is that you need to develop core stability to balance while doing those sit-ups and leg extensions. One of the hardest workouts we've ever had was on a ball. They come with a nifty small air pump, so you can take the ball when you travel. The balls cost in the range of $30 to $40. Excellent videos for the fitness ball range from easy and slow to highly challenging. Some videos for the fitness ball are great for aerobic/cardio conditioning. Fitness ball classes are also offered at many fitness centers.

> **Thinspiration**
>
> Strength-building exercises deliver quick visible results. As you continue to build muscle strength, the results only get better. Within six months of two sessions a week, you'll enjoy how your clothes look on you and how you feel.

◆ **Fitness circle.** This equipment has a 1-inch band of steel wrapped three times to form a circle, or ring, about 18 inches in diameter plus handles. You use the circle for resistance, such as doing a very slow sit-up while squeezing it between your knees. By using any one of the many videos or DVDs available on the fitness circle, you can have a complete and comprehensive strength and stretching session in 30 minutes. It can be packed in a suitcase. Cost varies from $20 on up, but the $20 version works well.

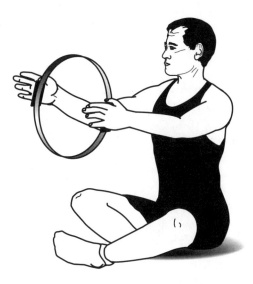

The fitness circle lets you gain stronger muscles as you do Pilates exercises.

The fitness ball, flex band, and fitness circle are equipment used in Pilates and other types of exercises. Check out Appendix B for information on where to purchase videos for this equipment. If you like using this list of simple equipment and you really fall in love with the elegant Pilates exercise system, you can go full out and purchase the Pilates Reformer.

> **Thinspiration** _____
>
> Check out Pilates-based exercises. Pilates, based on strength and flexibility techniques that Joseph Pilates taught to classical dancers beginning in the 1930s, is the hottest exercise approach sweeping the country. We predict it will be here long after other fads have passed on. The results you'll enjoy are most likely in line with how you want to look: strong, long, lean muscles and better posture. Many people even say they've gotten taller from doing Pilates! Find out for yourself. Check out your local phone book or health clubs near you for a beginner class or lesson.

All Pilates strength-building exercises require you to participate actively—by focusing on your body and concentrating on your form. This has a way of making Pilates very relaxing because it's impossible to worry about or even think about much else when you're doing it. The intense focus actually assists you in getting the full benefit from Pilates exercises. An added plus is that you don't sweat much, but you still get the strength and flexibility results you want.

Flexibility

Can you easily bend over to touch your toes? Can you sit cross-legged on the floor? If not, your body lacks flexibility. Having a flexible body is such a treat. It gives your movements grace and fluidity. You look great. Your spine is strong, and you're less likely to risk injury.

You gain flexibility from stretching exercises that elongate the body muscles. Stretching feels good. It's typically relaxing because, as you stretch, you release the tension held in your muscles.

We need to talk for a moment here about your tummy. If you're finding that all the abdominal crunches in the world aren't giving you a flat tummy, try stretching. Do a slow backbend over a fitness ball, stretching each part of the front of the body as you slowly roll back over the ball. Then turn over face down and stretch your back. This elongates your abdominal muscles and feels great.

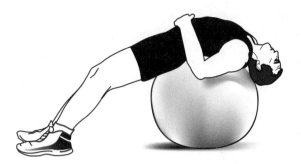

*Recline over the FitBall®
for an excellent abdominal
stretch.*

Here are some forms of exercise that will
help you stretch:

♦ Pilates

♦ Yoga

♦ Tibetans

♦ Flexibility and stretching classes

♦ Stretching videos and books

We suggest that you also stretch after your
cardio workouts and after strength training. In
fact, stretch every day just for the utter joy of it.

Thinspiration

Stretching is almost guaranteed
to make you feel better, and
you don't need to naturally be
a human pretzel to enjoy it. If
you're out of shape, stretching
exercises will pay off right away.
You'll learn to feel how your
body works, will begin to elongate your muscles, and will feel
more relaxed.

Combination Programs

You can combine more than one type of exercise at the same time in several different
ways. Dancing, karate, Tae Bo, and martial arts offer you various combinations of
cardio/aerobic, flexibility, and strength training. If you want to take up one of these
activities, what better time than now?

Get Out and Recreate

Cardio, strength, and flexibility are the basics for exercise, but let's not get too serious
and forget that there are lots of great ways to exercise when you're also having fun.
So recreate, okay? Find a friend or family member who would enjoy doing recreational activities with you. Couples and families that enjoy recreational exercise

together are healthier and do a better job of staying at their ideal size. Here's a partial list of recreational activities that feature great exercise:

- Dancing or dance lessons
- Biking
- Tennis
- Kayaking
- Racquetball

- Running/walking races
- Squash
- Walkathons
- Soccer
- Snow shoeing

- Hiking
- Skiing
- Cross-country skiing
- Swimming

Thinspiration

Lucy's hiking for recreation: "As my body adapted to mountain hiking, I experienced hiking as the perfect date with my husband. We now either hike or snowshoe most weekends. We pack along books on wildflowers and birds. We love being out in the clear air. And we especially enjoy doing it together. Hiking is so utterly exhilarating. It feels good all over."

Sandy's dancing classes for recreation: "My husband and I take weekly dance classes as a way to handle being empty-nesters. Now we have a regular dance 'date' every week and enjoy the movement and fun together. Nothing gets in the way of our dance date."

A Daily Dose of Five Essential Exercises

Years ago, in 1939, a small book titled *Ancient Secret of the Fountain of Youth* was published. Written by Peter Keldor, it told the story of an aging colonel who went to Tibet and returned 10 years later, looking many years younger. The colonel attributed his youthful appearance to doing these five exercises every day. They're affectionately known as the Tibetans.

The Tibetans get your heart pumping, although not long enough for full cardio benefits. They strengthen your muscles and improve your flexibility. Even better, they give you a great lift, like you had a cup of coffee without the coffee.

The five Tibetans have been passed around quietly for years, and those of us who do them routinely would never stop. Why? Because they deliver. After you've done the five Tibetan exercises for about three months, you'll notice you no longer have a double chin. It has vanished. Women eventually discover that their midriffs are sort of slinkier, and men often have lost several belt sizes ... even without losing weight.

The reported benefits of the Tibetans are as follows:

♦ Double chin gone

♦ Midriff slimmer

♦ Upper arms firmer

♦ More energy

♦ Increased muscle tone

♦ Early morning wake-up lift

The following is what researchers say the five Tibetans do for the body:

♦ Stimulate the reticular activating system of the brain.

♦ Balance the right and left hemispheres of the brain, which means you think more clearly. (You should definitely do the Tibetans before an exam or an important presentation!)

♦ Balance the body's hormonal system.

♦ Strengthen bones, as the exercises are weight-bearing.

♦ Improve the body's immune system.

♦ Build muscle strength.

♦ Reduce body-fat percentage.

♦ Boost metabolism.

♦ Align and strengthen the spine, plus make it more supple.

♦ Lighten menopausal symptoms.

♦ Lessen premenstrual symptoms.

♦ Help relieve the discomfort of arthritis and other aches and pains.

> **Thinspiration**
>
> On my 45th birthday, I, Lucy, received a copy of *Ancient Secrets of the Fountain of Youth* from my 19-year-old son. He gave me the book because, as he said, "Mom, you're getting old." Since that time, I have done the five simple Tibetan exercises faithfully every morning as I start my day. In just 5 to 10 minutes, I'm ready to take on whatever the day brings.

While Joe was on an extended business trip to London, he began doing the Tibetans two times a day, morning and late afternoon. He was careful to eat an amount of food the size of his fist three times a day. Plus he walked a lot. By the time he returned home to Australia, Joe had lost 4 inches around his waist. His wife didn't recognize him when he appeared at the front door. Joe was 56 years old.

Doing the Tibetans

We recommend that you do the Tibetans every morning when you wake up. They're easiest to do on an empty stomach. If the exercises seem too strenuous at first, refer to the book *Ancient Secrets of the Fountain of Youth, Part 2*, published by Doubleday, for starter exercises so that you can slowly build up strength to do the full recommended set.

For beginners, just start with three or four repetitions of each exercise for the first week. Then increase the number of repetitions by a few every week until you reach the full 21 repetitions. Do the repetitions of each exercise before moving on to the next exercise. If you never work all the way up to 21 each, don't worry; they will still deliver results.

The five Tibetan exercises can be performed anytime and virtually anywhere. It isn't necessary to do each exercise more than 21 times to receive all their benefits.

The Tibetans

Exercise 1: Standing with arms extended outward to the sides at shoulder height, spin your body toward your right hand. Go slowly at first and be sure to stop if you feel dizzy. Should you get dizzy, pick a spot on the wall and look at it until you feel clear-headed. Eventually, you will be able to spin quickly without getting dizzy. In the beginning, just spin three complete rotations, eventually working up to 21.

Spinning seems like an odd exercise, and in a way it is. But it wakes your body up and seems to stimulate proper hormonal balance. There's a reason why children love to spin—because it feels good and it's good for you.

Exercise 2: First lie flat on the floor, face up. Fully extend your arms along your sides and place the palms of your hands against the floor, keeping the fingers close together. If you want, place your hands under your hips to brace your movement. Then raise your head off the floor, tucking the chin against the chest. As you do this, lift your legs, knees straight, into a vertical position, perpendicular to the floor. If possible, let the legs extend back over the body toward the head, but do not let the knees bend. Then slowly lower both your head and legs, knees straight, to the floor. Breathe in deeply as you lift your legs and breathe out as you lower your legs.

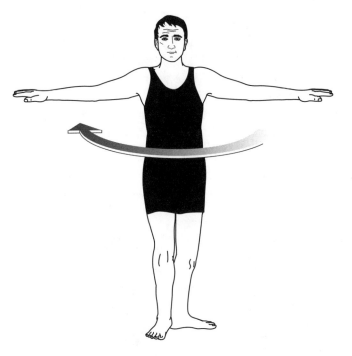

Exercise 1.

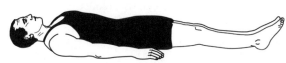

Exercise 2.

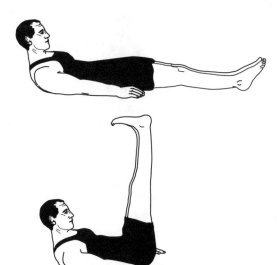

Exercise 3: Kneel on the floor with the torso of your body erect. Place your hands behind your back either in the middle back or lower back. Bend your neck and head forward, tucking the chin against the chest. Then move the head and neck backward slowly, arching your spine. As you arch, you brace your hands against your body for support. Go backward until you are looking up at the ceiling and your neck feels fully stretched. After the arching, return to the original position and start the second repetition. Breathe in deeply as you arch the spine and breathe out as you return to an erect position.

Exercise 3.

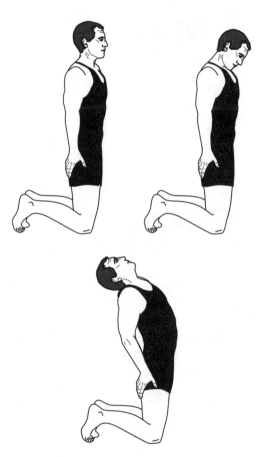

Exercise 4: Sit down on the floor with your legs straight out in front of you and your feet about 12 inches apart. Sit up straight and place the palms of your hands on the floor alongside your buttocks, fingers pointed toward your toes. Tuck your chin forward against the chest. Then slowly drop your head backward as far as it will go. At

the same time, raise your body so that the knees bend while the arms remain straight. The only body parts touching the floor are the palms of your hands and the soles of your feet.

The trunk of your body will be aligned with the upper legs, horizontal to the floor. Your body will be in the shape of a bench. Then tense every muscle in the body. Finally, relax your muscles as you return to the original sitting position and rest before repeating the procedure. Breathe in as you raise up, hold your breath as you tense the muscles, and breathe out completely as you come down.

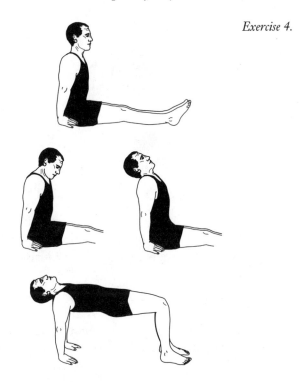

Exercise 4.

Exercise 5: When you perform the fifth exercise, your body is facing the floor with just your toes and hands on the floor. Make a tent shape out of your body, with your head tucked between your arms and your bottom up. Then move your torso toward the floor so that you are flexing the spine in reverse and look up at the ceiling. Breathe in deeply as you raise your body and breathe out fully as you lower it.

Exercise 5.

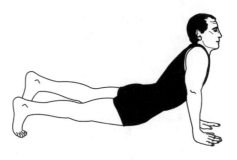

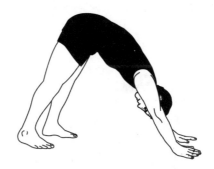

The five Tibetans are an exercise "extra" to boost your fitness progress. They're a great way to start the day, and they fit nicely with other parts of your exercise program. Clients rave about the results they get. You'll love the results, too.

The Least You Need to Know

- There are three kinds of exercise—aerobic/cardio, strength training, and stretching—that you should do to feel good, look good, stay healthy, and reach your ideal size.

- Choose the exercise approaches you like the best and that work for you and your family.

- Include regular recreational exercise for fun, variety, and the joy of the activity.

- Do the five Tibetans every day upon waking; they feel good and do great things for you and your body.

21

Design Your Personal Exercise Plan

In This Chapter

- ◆ Choosing a personal exercise approach
- ◆ Setting exercise goals
- ◆ Overcoming exercise obstacles
- ◆ Keeping yourself motivated

By now you may be thinking, "How do I get all this exercise done and still have a life?" Or you might be wondering whether the trick to weight loss is to exercise so much that you don't even have time to eat!

In this chapter, we'll show you how to design a program that works for you and that you can use with confidence. We want you to truly enjoy exercising, so it's important to figure out an approach that's just right for you.

Your Comfort Zone

The first thing you need to figure out is where you want to exercise. You'll want to feel comfortable about your selected place. You basically have three choices for day-in, day-out exercise: home, the *gym*, or both. You need to figure out which suits your lifestyle best and helps you stay on track. Each has advantages and disadvantages.

Lean Lingo

Think of a **gym** as any place designed for exercise, such as a health club, a fitness center, a specialty studio, or a local recreational center. If you haven't been in a health club recently, the range of equipment and classes available might surprise you. You'll discover sophisticated exercise equipment, tennis or racquet courts, personal trainers, aerobic classes, Pilates instruction, yoga classes, and many other exercise offerings.

Benefits of at-home exercising:

♦ It may be more convenient for your schedule.

♦ You don't need to get dressed up.

♦ The shower is readily available.

♦ You don't need to drive anywhere.

♦ Instruction is available through excellent videos available today.

♦ You can hire a personal trainer to come to your home.

♦ You can use television or Internet exercise programs.

♦ It's efficient because you don't have travel time.

Drawbacks of at-home exercising:

♦ It requires lots of self-discipline.

♦ You are subject to distractions and interruptions from family members and the phone.

♦ Is not social. (This can be either good or bad, depending on your preference.)

♦ It may require you to purchase equipment.

♦ It requires floor space to exercise.

Benefits of exercising at a gym:

◆ Professional, varied classes and groups.

◆ The opportunity to meet other people.

◆ Group motivation.

◆ Professional-quality exercise equipment.

◆ Encouragement to push yourself harder.

◆ Extra motivation because you are paying for it.

◆ Often offer courts for racquetball, tennis, or volleyball.

◆ May offer indoor running and walking tracks.

◆ May have swimming pool with lanes for aerobic swimmers.

◆ Personal trainers on hand for consultations.

Drawbacks of exercising at a gym:

◆ The hassle of getting there via car or other transportation.

◆ You might need to adapt your schedule to their classes.

◆ The monthly cost needs to be factored into your household budget.

◆ The possible awkwardness of exercising in public.

◆ Non-private locker rooms.

Even if you join a gym, it's important to have a backup plan for exercising at home. Use it when you can't get to the gym or when you're traveling or on vacation. Yes, you hear us correctly. Just because you can't get to the gym is absolutely no excuse for missing your personal exercise appointment with yourself.

Thinspiration

If you're a woman and new to working out at an exercise facility, check out circuit training studios, such as Contours Express. They offer 30-minute fitness routines that combine aerobics and strength training with specially designed woman-sized weight machines that let you add more weight resistance as you grow stronger. You'll receive a personalized program along with knowledgeable and sincere support.

The Exercise Appointment

Do you use some form of calendar or appointment book? Or do you just keep a schedule in your head? In either case, make a date to exercise. At the beginning of every week, schedule your exercise appointments into your daily planner. Give yourself enough time for travel, exercise, and showering. An hour class could take two hours or more when you factor in the whole experience.

Every exercise appointment you set is a commitment to yourself. Keep your exercise appointments as sacred as a date with your spouse, attending ballgames using your season tickets, or business meetings. Don't make excuses for breaking the dates with yourself. The price is too high. We wish there were an easier way, but there just isn't an alternative to exercising.

For about a year, Debra attended a Bikram yoga class four to five times a week. This form of yoga was developed by Bikram Choudhury in Los Angeles and is now taught widely in the United States. It consists of 26 poses done in a room heated to about 100 degrees. The class itself was one and a half hours long. Travel each way was about 35 minutes. But to get a spot in the front near the mirror so that she could watch her postural alignment, Debra arrived a half-hour before class started. Yes, her yoga class took more than three hours! Fortunately, it was a great class for her and was well worth the time invested. Eventually, her lifestyle changed, with more responsibilities and obligations, and today, she couldn't begin to commit that much time so often. She still exercises daily, but now it's at home, at a local fitness center, or outdoors.

Don't count on "making up" missed exercise appointments. They often never get done for one reason or another. If you're a person who simply doesn't schedule yourself well, perhaps you need to schedule twice as many exercise dates so that you can meet your commitment to yourself. Remember that, with exercise, you aren't accountable to anyone else—only to yourself and your body.

Schedule the time of day that works best for you. If you're not a morning person, planning to be at the gym by 6 A.M. just isn't going to work for long. Perhaps you would enjoy exercising right after work before you go home. Set your appointments for the time of day that works for you. You might also want to break up the time. For example, do 20 minutes or more of aerobics in the morning before you get in the shower; then do your strength training later in the day.

You hardly need to schedule time to do the five Tibetans because they only take 5 minutes (or 10 minutes at most). We figure that doing them should be about as ordinary and routine as brushing your teeth. You just do them.

What to Do

No matter which forms of exercise you choose, here are the minimum amounts you should plan on in a week. By "minimum," we mean the very least you need. However, with exercise—unlike with food—more is often better.

Here is a guideline:

◆ Aerobics: 20 minutes daily or 45 minutes three times a week

◆ Strength: 45 minutes to an hour twice a week

◆ Stretching: 15 to 30 minutes twice a week or more

With exercise, you can vary the routine, learn new ones, and never get bored. Exercise is one area in your life where you can include an almost unlimited number of variations. You're not stuck with just one approach. You can add lots of fun activities to your basic exercise program. These add-ons are, in a sense, "free" treats. There may not be any free foods, but there sure is free exercise. So, yes, limit foods but don't limit your exercise. You can fill your "dance card" with fun movement and exercise. In this case, more is better and better for you. Plan on enjoying exercise and recreation so much that you prefer them to just sitting around or rushing around. Your body will thank you.

On the Road

As we said earlier, there are no excuses for not exercising, and that includes business travel and vacations. You don't give up food when you travel, so why would you give up exercise?

Many enlightened hotels and motels have exercise rooms with enough equipment to get your endorphins lifted and your heart rate elevated for 20 minutes or so. If not, get creative. Do step-ups on the staircase at equipment-deficient hotels. Yes, it looks weird to the people using the stairs (usually very few folks), but looking weird is better than not exercising.

We know there's a floor in your room, and a floor is all you need to do the five Tibetans. Some hotel rooms have VCRs or

Thinspiration

Treat exercise on the road as you would eating on the road—make it essential. You'll find that it increases your energy and makes your trip more enjoyable.

DVDs on which you can play a favorite exercise video. Plus, you can view exercise videos on DVD on your laptop.

Some equipment is easy to pack, such as a fitness circle, a fitness ball, or an elastic exercise band. Use these to get in your strength training. We know people who take free weights on the road, but that's beyond the scope of what we're willing to lug through airports.

Exercise-Altering Conditions

Other things can happen to interrupt your exercise plans. Let's discuss these and find solutions.

Weather

Weather happens. Yucky weather can keep you from walking, jogging, hiking, or swimming. It can even keep you from getting to the gym if the roads are icy. Make sure that you have alternative plans. In-home exercising is the obvious solution. Be clever, be smart, and don't let rain, sleet, or snow keep you from your exercise.

Ailments

If you have a seasonal cold or flu, exercise actually can stimulate your immune system and aid your recovery. But be careful not to overdo it. Low-impact activities such as yoga and Pilates are good choices, so you don't need to stay in bed unless the doctor orders it.

> **Weighty Warning**
>
> If you're in pretty good shape, your body will recover faster after surgery. But don't rush it. After an emergency appendectomy, Lucy needed two weeks before she could even try the Tibetans. And then it took another two weeks before she could do them all fully. The good news was that her everyday commitment to fitness helped her recover more quickly.

Following surgery, take your time to recover. As soon as you can, though, start moving and do as much as you can without injuring yourself. Get your doctor's advice on how soon you can exercise.

Bodily aches can certainly make exercise unpleasant, and yet the benefits might actually help. Even those suffering from terrible arthritis are encouraged to exercise as much as possible. Check with your doctor and with a sports therapist for what you can do within your current limitations. Often you have plenty of options.

Sports Injuries

Unfortunately, sports injuries sometimes result from exercise. Should this happen, of course, rest and rehabilitate. You might need to learn new ways of movement so that you can avoid injuries in the future. Most sports rehab involves movement and gradually rebuilding your strength, so you can continue to exercise. Be sure to include stretching in your weekly program.

Pregnancy

Yes, you can exercise when pregnant, just carefully. Be sure to check with your doctor before you begin. Then join an exercise class designed for pregnant women or use one of the videos especially for this time of your life.

Setting Goals

Our favorite adage about goals is to start slowly and to go quickly. Way too often, new exercisers have great expectations about their bodies. Then they pay the price for overdoing it. How about you?

Have you ever gone to an aerobics class at the gym and tried really hard to keep up with the person in front of you? You got an A+ for effort. You gasped for breath, and your legs shook from the exertion, but you soldiered on. The next morning and the following day, your body ached unmercifully. Simple activities such as walking and going up stairs seemed next to impossible. Boy, were you asking for it!

If this happens to you, try the following to recover the next day: stretching sore muscles, hot Epsom salts baths, Emergen-C to replenish electrolytes, and massage to remove lactic acid from muscles.

Start slowly. Gradually increase your exercise time or intensity to allow your body to adapt. Work up gradually to 20 minutes of cardio/aerobics. Ditto strength training. Ditto stretching.

> **Thinspiration**
>
> A personal goal helps. Your goal might be to attain an acceptable level of aerobics and maintain it. Your goal might be to climb Mount Everest. Perhaps you want to take up a particular sport or outdoor activity. For most of us, though, just getting in shape, staying in shape, and having fun doing it are plenty.

You can always modify your goals if you want more, and there can be good reasons to want more. You might have a specific objective on which you want to focus. For example, we find that strength training is more helpful to fit into your clothes at 40 or 50 or even 60 years old. Plus the bone-strengthening factor of strength training becomes more significant with age.

The Scorecard

Your most important scorecard is how you look and feel, plus how you fit into your clothes. Another important scorecard is how your mood and perspective are lifted as you continue your cardio/aerobics, strengthening, and flexibility program.

We also realize that keeping a tally sheet helps. A rule of thumb in business is that what you count tends to increase. The same is true of exercise. If you count clicks on a pedometer, you'll most likely jog or run more. If you count exercise sessions, you tend to do more of them. With that in mind, we suggest that you keep a weekly and monthly exercise chart.

Weekly Exercise Scorecard

	Cardio/Aerobic	Strength-Training	Flexibility
	Method Duration	*Method Duration*	*Method Duration*
Monday			
Tuesday			
Wednesday			
Thursday			
Friday			
Saturday			
Sunday			
Total for week			

Put a copy of your scorecard on your desk or in your daily planner. Perhaps tape it to your bathroom mirror. At the end of the week, review how well you did.

Exercise is vital to reaching your ideal size and staying there for life. It gives you energy, soothes stress, and boosts your metabolism. The higher your metabolism, the easier it is to lose weight and keep it off. The less stress you experience, the less stress eating you'll do. Plus, the more energy you have, the easier it is to eat from 0–5.

Thinspiration

When you review your exercise scorecard, if you didn't do as well as you planned, don't become upset with yourself. Forgive yourself and do better the next week, but don't quit keeping score because you'll lessen your resolve.

The Least You Need to Know

◆ Decide whether you are better off exercising at home or at a gym, based on how each fits with your lifestyle and personality.

◆ Make sure that you have an at-home program for the days when you can't get to the gym or when you are on the road.

◆ Keep up your exercise program during vacations and business travel.

◆ Have realistic goals for making progress and continuing the program for life.

◆ Keep track of your fitness progress by using a diary, scorecard, or fitness log.

Part 6

Understanding Weight-Loss Plans

Every day, almost everywhere, you're bombarded with advertisements, articles, and hype on the latest diet plan or weight-loss system. Few of them offer lasting results. Most offer hope when you're feeling desperate on a chubby Monday morning. Some offer a chance to lose a couple of pounds quickly but little else. Of course, the weight is back the next week. A couple of approaches to weight loss are real gems. They might just work for you. In this part of the book, we review popular diet plans and show you how to find the jewels amid the hype.

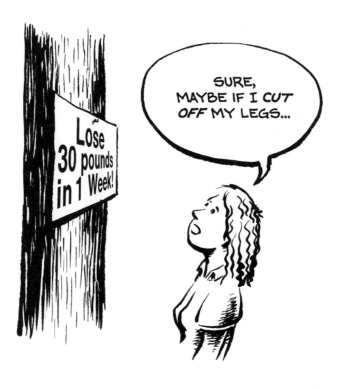

Chapter 22

Rating Popular Diet Programs

In This Chapter

- ◆ Evaluating time-tested weight-loss programs
- ◆ Using criteria for selecting any program
- ◆ Understanding the problems with prepackaged diet foods
- ◆ Getting the most from the Internet

Diets of one kind or another are still going strong. Although our Paleolithic ancestors probably didn't fret over extra pounds, that's certainly not true in modern times. Diets have been around throughout the twentieth century and now into the twenty-first century. You can be pretty sure they'll still be around in the next century, too.

Since at least the 1950s, Americans have turned to others for help in shedding pounds and keeping them off. We've wanted someone to give us a "plan" that will do the trick. Hence, today there are many weight-loss programs offered at studios and storefront locations. And yes, they've guided many people to their ideal size, at least for a while, and some for life.

There's much good to be said for popular weight-loss programs. Most of the time, they're sensible and focus on your lifelong quest to reach and stay at your ideal size. Typically, their meal plans are pretty balanced, with an emphasis on the eating guidelines of the classic food pyramid. Today, several of these plans have updated themselves and introduced terrific websites that support their users.

Unfortunately, just because some weight-loss programs have been around for decades, it doesn't mean they're right for you. We think some of them have real problems. Let's take a closer look.

Buy Our Food, Lose Weight ... Right?

Some of the best-known *diet systems* offer prepackaged foods. Why? Because you need help. Right? Out of desperation, you don't even want to think about what and how to eat. "Just tell me what to do!" you cry out.

Prepackaged foods are touted as the ideal convenience. They offer portion control and the "right" kinds of food. On the surface, it makes perfectly good sense that you would turn to someone to tell you what to eat because you haven't succeeded on you own. Plus, these systems also offer various kinds of psychological support to make your new eating regimen more palatable.

Let's look at how well these systems might or might not work for you in attaining and maintaining your ideal size for life while eating for health and energy.

Weight Watchers

Weight Watchers is practically a household name. The company has been in business for about 45 years and is most famous for its weekly weigh-in meetings. At these meetings, members weigh themselves in a group setting, receiving "hurrahs!" from other members when they show progress and lots of emotional support when they don't.

Lean Lingo

A weight-loss program, sometimes known as a **diet system,** is primarily an organized eating plan to assist you in losing weight and keeping it off. Typically, they offer very specific suggestions for what foods to eat, how often to eat, portion control, and other eating "rules." Some of the best-known plans offer their own prepackaged foods or special supplements.

Weighty Warning

You can get to your ideal size and stay there for life by eating regular everyday ordinary foods. Special diet foods are not the answer to your weight-loss problems. Be sure that any plan you choose stands on its own without "diet" foods or shakes.

As Weight Watchers has grown, it has added a monthly magazine, processed foods and meals that are available in grocery stores, and a website that's useful and informative.

Weight Watchers brand prepackaged food might offer portion control, but it's far from ideal. It overemphasizes low fat and is high-glycemic. Plus, it's loaded with heavily processed foods and preservatives. Not good. We don't recommend that you eat Weight Watchers food products. Fortunately, you don't have to. You can still take advantage of the weekly support groups.

Weight Watchers has dramatically revised its recommended eating plan. There was a time when each member weighed and measured all food and could only eat so much of certain types of foods at every meal. It was a very regimented eating system.

Today, Weight Watchers uses a point system, and they also offer a core program if a person doesn't want to count. For the point system, based on a person's desired weight and other factors, each member is given a certain number of points to eat each day. This way, a person can have a piece of cake or ice cream and still lose weight. So far, so good. You can choose the best ratios of protein, fats, and carbs for you. We also like this.

Weight Watchers designates some foods as "free foods," meaning you can eat them whenever you want with no limit to quantity. Typically, free foods are raw vegetables such as celery, cabbage, and radishes. Just be sure that if you use this program, you don't overeat "free foods." Otherwise, you'll still be abusing your body with too much food.

One of our concerns with Weight Watchers is that you can get too hungry! Nancy was a member of Weight Watchers who thought she would like the simple "organization" of a point system. But most days she ate all her points for the day by noon. From noon on, she wouldn't eat again until the next morning. At dinner, she would sit with her family while they ate the dinner she cooked. Sure, she could eat a plate full of celery while they ate a robust meal, but that seemed less appealing than not eating at all … especially after the fourth or fifth day! One day Nancy realized that the unconscious messages she was sending to her family, especially her teenaged daughter, were not healthy.

Many serious eating disorders, such as bulimia and anorexia, are rooted in a parent's conscious and unconscious messages to the child about weight and eating. Nancy was silently telling her daughter that it was okay to put her body into extreme hunger for the sake of sticking to her diet (and that it was okay to follow rigid eating rituals). Nancy didn't want her daughter to emulate her eating and develop both weight and eating issues, so she quit the program.

Thinspiration

Food isn't the enemy. Any diet system that causes you to "starve" yourself during even part of the day creates an unhealthy attitude about eating. Food itself becomes evil, and all foods become "forbidden fruit." Often this leads to starvation metabolism and subsequent binge eating.

Body of Knowledge

Some formal weight-loss programs are great for delivering motivation and support. They can help you stay on course and avoid discouragement, but don't let the regimentation or poor nutritional advice interfere with your healthy and commonsense approach to food and eating.

Weight Watchers seems to move a bit slowly in response to current nutritional research. But recently it's started recommending nutrient-dense health foods in both its core and point systems. It subscribes to a low-fat, calorie-controlled eating approach and now encourages members to get plenty of essential fatty acids every day.

That said, the support system is very helpful. You can even "go to meetings" online, which means you can save your evenings for family and fun. We like this.

Weight Watchers strongly encourages exercise and does a great job of showing members how to put together home programs.

Its maintenance program is challenging to stick with, as is any maintenance plan. As with all dieters who rebound from restricted calorie intake, a member's tendency is to go overboard and make up for lost time. Easing into normal eating is quite challenging and not as successful as the original weight-loss results.

If you choose to use Weight Watchers, we encourage you to always eat 0–5 and not be tempted to overeat free foods. Avoid the company's prepackaged meals and foods. Take your essential fatty acids every day and avoid high-glycemic starches. Eat at least 40 grams of high-quality protein every day. Weight Watchers's support and exercise suggestions are great.

Evaluating Other Weight-Loss Programs

Just look in your local phone book to find many more weight-loss centers and programs. Before you visit them, call and ask the following questions to determine whether you should even consider visiting. The sales reps will often urge you to come in and talk because they know how to sell you when you are there in person. It's hard to ask analytical questions after the box of Kleenex comes out, and you're in the throes of emotion. So resist the sales rep's urging and try to get answers to these questions over the phone before you visit:

Question	Preferred Answer
Do you offer prepackaged foods, and do I need to eat them?	No, we want you to eat your own food.
Do I have to weigh?	No.
Does the plan encourage or discourage me from skipping meals or not eating for periods of time?	We discourage any kind of starvation mode. We make sure you get adequate food on a day-to-day basis to keep your metabolism and energy high.
Do you recommend low-glycemic eating?	Yes, we do.
What percentage fat do you recommend?	Between 25–30%.
Do you recommend that I take essential fatty acids?	Yes, EFAs will help you burn excess fat.
Do you recommend I use a hunger scale?	Yes, we want you to learn how to know your body and honor its hunger needs.
Is there a maintenance plan?	The plan you'll use to get to your ideal size is basically the same one you'll use to stay there.
Do you suggest I use any products containing ephedra, bitter orange, ma huang, or country mallow? (More information on these products in Chapter 11.)	No, for health reasons, we don't promote their use.
Do you suggest I use bulking agents so that I feel full?	No, we don't use them.
Does your program include soy shakes or protein drinks?	No, our program doesn't. You can use them occasionally if you want.
Do you recommend an exercise program?	Yes, we'll help you design one that suits you and your lifestyle.
How fast can I lose my weight?	We don't encourage fast weight loss but rather genuine, slow loss that stays off. We know the dangers of yo-yo dieting and want you to avoid it.
Do you recommend that I use artificial sweeteners such as aspartame, weak saccharine, or Splenda?	No.
Can you give me the names of several people who have used your system? I would like to call them. I want to talk with a couple of people who were successful, and some who were not.	We don't give out client names, but we can ask several to phone you.

Only after a weight-loss program answers these questions to your satisfaction should you consider setting up a meeting. When you do go, stay alert. Consider other alternatives and don't sign anything on your first visit.

CAUTION

Weighty Warning

Before you visit a weight-loss program or diet center, pause and ask yourself why you're going. Is it for motivational support? If so, maybe the program will help. Or is it because you can't control your own eating and need to be forced into a rigid plan? If so, the weight-loss system might not be adequate to help you stay at your ideal size for life. You might be setting yourself up for one more yo-yo dieting failure.

Overeaters Anonymous

Overeaters Anonymous is a not-for-profit organization that offers support groups to assist people who are overweight and obese. Their premise is that overeating is an addiction and a disease. The program uses a 12-step approach adapted from Alcoholics Anonymous.

The meetings are free with donations welcome. You can attend as many meetings as you want. Overeaters Anonymous encourages members to avoid sugars and other designated "addictive" foods. They support balanced meals and wholesome nutrition.

The addiction and disease model works well for overeating and works well for some people who binge-eat regularly. And avoiding sugars and fluffy starches—the high-glycemic starches—is always a good plan. An alcoholic can abstain forever from drinking; however, a person can't abstain from eating. At each meeting, visitors introduce themselves by saying, "My name is (*state first name only*), and I am a compulsive overeater."

Thinspiration

Please don't ever call yourself a "compulsive overeater." Instead, affirm your positive self-image. Say, "I am now at my ideal size. I easily master my weight and my eating." You'll learn more about affirmations in Part 6.

Therein lies our biggest problem with Overeaters Anonymous. We don't believe that after a person is a compulsive overeater, he or she is forever a compulsive overeater. Although overeating often involves powerful underlying psychological issues, we don't believe overeating should be classified the same as alcoholism.

Studies show that what a person thinks and says is usually a self-fulfilling prophecy. Certainly, the spiritual focus at the group meetings is valuable, and the group support can be terrific. But overall, we suggest you use a more positively affirming program.

Web-Based Eating Plans

The web and weight loss are quickly becoming linked. It's really quite exciting how you can now use the Internet to assist you with weight loss. Even though the web as a tool for weight loss is relatively new, it offers some powerful new approaches. For instance, by first surveying your vital statistics and food preferences, you can get a customized eating plan. Plus, you can get support and information online. Some of the weight-loss sites are great. But watch out, some are really bad.

Watch Out for E-Miracles

By now, you and everyone else with a web connection have received unsolicited e-mails promoting the latest diet craze. Talk about the weight-loss promised land! Whew! You're offered "guaranteed" miracles to shed pounds effortlessly. All you need to do is send cash. Yes, some say, only send cash. Oh, come on. If any of these e-mail solicitations had discovered a miracle approach for weight loss, you'd be reading about it in the newspapers and seeing it on *60 Minutes*. Please don't send them money. The promoters know you're vulnerable because you could be desperate to lose weight.

The Really Good Web-Based Programs

Now for the good web-based weight-loss programs. As of the time of this writing, there were several. You might discover others in your web searching. We like these:

- ◆ eDiets
- ◆ CyberDiets
- ◆ iVillage

> **Body of Knowledge**
>
> You can find registered dietitians who counsel on the web by doing a search for the keyword "dietitian." You can also go to the American Dietetic Association site at www.eatright.org to find a dietitian located near you.

They generally offer a balanced and sensible approach. Many are free, and if not, the cost is minimal. They offer chat rooms for support and exercise recommendations. Some even chart your progress for you. They might offer recommended eating plans and caloric intake, but because the plans are driven by formulas built into their programming, you'll need to determine whether the plan really makes sense for you. The good sites use registered dietitians for counseling and information. They send frequent e-mail newsletters for news and encouragement.

We like many of the sites because they help you deal with stress and emotional eating. Just think, when you want to eat when you aren't hungry, you can just go online and get instant support! You don't need to wait for a friend to return your calls—just get online.

As you check out weight-loss websites, look for the ones that feel good to you. Some web-based weight-loss sites might make recommendations for eating based on formulas that aren't right for you. For instance, the formula might recommend a caloric intake that leaves you undernourished, perhaps sending you into starvation metabolism. Apply caution and common sense when using automated weight-loss plans. Use the info that makes sense to you and toss the rest. Remember, only you know what works for your body.

The Least You Need to Know

- If you want to use a packaged diet system, make sure that it meets your standards.

- Avoid eating prepackaged diet foods; they're typically high-glycemic, highly processed, and often too low in fat.

- Emotional support and encouragement, plus exercise coaching, are often the better features of weight-loss programs.

- Take advantage of Internet sites for weight-loss support.

- Just delete those unsolicited e-mails for the newest miracle weight-loss products.

Chapter 23

Food and Eating Philosophies

In This Chapter

- A "fast" way to lose weight
- Vegetarianism and weight loss
- Other philosophical eating approaches
- Eating concepts that better fit your biological needs

Throughout the ages, food has served cultural purposes that go beyond sustenance and pleasure. In many religions, rituals and rules cover many aspects of eating. Some religions restrict certain kinds of foods; some govern how food is prepared and when it can be eaten.

In some religions, food—or fasting from food—is used for ritual purification or as a way to seek higher levels of holiness. For many ages, food has been considered a source for healing and for boosting energy and longevity.

Philosophical approaches to eating add an extra layer—and sometimes extra pounds—to the challenge of reaching your ideal size. Today, many people use these methods for weight loss, although, in general, their origins had nothing to do with weight management. Remember, just because a food ritual has been used for religious reasons for hundreds of years doesn't automatically make it better nutritionally. In this chapter, we will explore both ancient and modern food philosophies.

Fasting

If your religion mandates that you fast as a spiritual practice, by all means, follow the precepts of your chosen religion. *Fasting* for spiritual reasons is a traditional part of the Catholic, Jewish, Hindu, and Muslim faiths, as well as many others. Most of these incorporate fasting as part of special rituals or religious holidays.

If you fast, we hope it is because you are following a traditional religion and not the modern day "religion" of dieting and weight loss. But if you're fasting as a way to lose weight or to control your weight, you might have noticed that it doesn't seem to be working. Let's talk about why.

Lean Lingo

Fasting is the act of abstaining from eating for a period of time, usually one or more days. Often a person ingests only water or juice during this time.

Fasting is usually done by avoiding solid or nutritive foods and some nutritive liquids. Water, or perhaps juice, is all that's allowed. By not eating when your body is hungry and by not eating balanced meals, even for a day, you put your body into starvation metabolism. In starvation metabolism, your body slows down metabolically and starts hoarding bodily fat so that you don't starve to death. As you learned earlier in the book, your biological programming for starvation metabolism is strong and resolute. Remember that the body doesn't know how long the fast is going to last, so it prepares for the worst. You know that the fast will last only a day or a couple of days, but your body doesn't.

Fasting is an especially tricky problem for the many overweight people who have low blood sugar. Going without food for longer than four to five hours makes them weak, nauseous, and irritable rather than energized and happy. For these folks, when the fast is finally over, they often binge-eat to recover from the deprivation and to feel better.

One well-meaning woman, Sylvia, like may others, believed that fasting was a good way to let her digestion rest, to detoxify her body, and to drop a couple of pounds. Her fasting was not based on the precepts of any religion to which she belonged. All she would allow herself was water and two glasses of orange juice for three days. To detoxify, however, the liver needs high-quality protein, the digestive system doesn't really need rest, and most of the pounds she lost were regained within a day or two after she resumed eating. Fruit juice just isn't comparable to high-quality protein and essential fatty acids.

Weighty Warning

Beware of using fasting as a weight-loss method. It isn't healthy and can cause more problems than you want to deal with, such as binge-eating and weight gain.

Sylvia was one of the many people who fast as a way to lose weight. They fast every month or so. Because fasters sometimes step on the scale at the end of the fast and see that a few pounds have been lost, they keep coming back. Not smart. Fasting to lose weight brings on unnecessary problems—starvation metabolism, weakness, binge-eating, and a return of the lost pounds. You should choose better ways to get to your ideal size.

We don't recommend fasting. In fact, we urge you to avoid fasting for weight loss. It isn't healthy.

Vegetarianism

Vegetarianism began as a religious practice many thousands of years ago. Here's how it all began. In hot climates, such as India, people who ate meat from hoofed animals, meaning cattle and pigs, often became painfully sick and died. When people ate fish and poultry, this didn't happen. Why? Because fish and chicken could be killed and prepared to feed a family for a particular meal. But a whole slaughtered cow or pig couldn't be eaten in one day. Since refrigeration was not available, the leftover meat putrefied quickly. The leftovers were poisonous, to say the least.

In colder climates, such as northern Europe and Asia and the Americas, meat could be safely eaten for several days because it was cold outside much of the year. Also, the indigenous people dried meat and fish—as in beef jerky—to eat later. In hot climates, the meat would have putrefied before it could be dried.

In India, as a way to keep people from eating the beef and pork, the priests and elders declared the cow to be sacred and the pig unclean. Over the years, these eating restrictions became incorporated into today's Hindu religion. Similar food restrictions became part of other religions in hot climates where the cow and pig were indigenous.

Modern-Day Vegetarianism

Vegetarianism today isn't the same. As you can see, religious vegetarianism was rooted in a practical, commonsense solution to a deadly situation. With today's refrigeration, these eating rules could be loosened, but since they're tied to established religious doctrine, that won't likely occur.

Vegetarianism today has almost become its own religion, with many varied sects. During the past several decades, many people have avoided meat as a path to holiness or higher spiritual experiences. Others avoid eating meat for personal ethical reasons, refusing to support the slaughter of four-legged animals for food. Others avoid meat because they believe it is unnatural or unhealthy to eat. For some, vegetarianism becomes wrapped up in their political views of the world. Unfortunately, many think it's a great way to lose weight. It's not.

Here are the five broad categories of vegetarians, with lots of personal variations:

- **Vegans** avoid all animal products (meaning meat, fish, poultry, eggs, milk, cheese, and other dairy products), even the wearing of leather shoes.

- **Nonmeat vegetarians** eat eggs, dairy, and fish, but not the meat from four-legged animals.

- **Lacto-vegetarians** avoid meat, poultry, fish, and eggs, but eat dairy products.

- **Ovo-lacto vegetarians** eat eggs and dairy products but not poultry, fish, or meat from other animals.

- **Semi-vegetarians** mostly follow a vegetarian plan with occasional intakes of meat, poultry, or fish.

Sometimes a person's choice is based on religious rules, sometimes on perceived health benefits, and sometimes on judgments about the ethical issues involved with killing certain kinds of animals for food.

Vegetarianism and Weight Loss

Strict vegetarianism as a lifestyle practice is fine, but don't expect it to be an enlightened path to weight loss. We see too many vegetarian clients with stubborn weight-loss problems to recommend it for losing weight. However, vegetarians who eat at least fish and fowl can get to their ideal size by eating the balanced food plan recommended in this book and by eating 0–5.

If a person's vegetarian preferences are more extreme, it's nearly impossible to lose weight and keep it off. Eating eggs and cheese can get truly boring, and you have to eat lots of them to get enough complete high-quality protein—like a couple dozen eggs a week and several pounds of cheese! We question the wisdom of this because of the lack of variety, plus constantly eating the same foods invites allergies.

> **Weighty Warning**
>
> Many vegetarians inadvertently become starcharians because instead of eating more vegetables, they end up eating more starches. Eating lots of starches is an easy way to pack on the pounds.

Vegans have an even tougher time losing weight. Vegans regularly fail to get enough complete high-quality protein, and they tend to eat lots of starches, which can really pack on the weight.

Sally was a member of the Hari Krishna religious group for more than seven years. With Hindu roots, the sect promotes strict vegetarianism. When I asked how she handled eating no meat for all those years, she replied, "I am a vegetarian in spirit and philosophy, but my body isn't. So I eat meat because my body needs it."

Many of our clients have found that when they add animal protein back into their diets, the weight comes off, and they can maintain their ideal size. If you are vegetarian and you can't lose weight, we strongly urge you to start introducing fish, poultry, and meat into your diet until you are eating about 15 to 20 grams of animal protein three times a day.

> **Weighty Warning**
>
> Total or complete vegetarians, vegans, often struggle with other health issues besides stubborn body fat. Often their hair, nails, night vision, and skin are less than healthy. Many complain of low energy, which often results in binge-eating to compensate. Sometimes supplements can offset the lost nutrients and micronutrients, but basically their bodies are craving high-quality protein.

Although we respect philosophical vegetarianism, we also believe that eating meat respects our human nature. Eating animal protein can also be an ethical, philosophical approach to food.

> **Thinspiration**
>
> In one of her many attempts to lose weight, Lucy adopted a totally vegetarian macrobiotic diet. She worked with a macrobiotic specialist who guided her food choices. After 4 months she had gained another 20 pounds, and her husband, who was already quite thin, lost about 20 pounds. Her four-year-old son, Brian, complained of being too tired to walk around the block. Lucy rushed him to the pediatrician.
>
> The diagnosis was anemia. When she told the pediatrician about the family's commitment to macrobiotic eating, he became enraged. Right there, in the waiting room, he loudly commanded her to stop at the grocery store on the way home, buy steaks and a cast iron skillet, and "feed her family and not ever let that child become anemic again."
>
> Within a month, Lucy's 20 pounds were gone, her husband got his weight back up, and her son was his normal—highly active—self. When Brian turned 16, he advised his mom that he was going to become a vegetarian. Her response was, "Over my dead body and yours." Then she told him about his earlier run-in with vegetarian-induced anemia. He changed his mind.
>
> Lucy's weight loss of 20 pounds in a month wasn't the result of going on a diet. Instead, the weight simply fell off when she got out of starvation metabolism.

The Blood-Type Philosophy

Can eating foods in harmony with your blood type assist you in losing weight? That's the premise of the blood-type diet. Proponents also claim that a person can eliminate allergies and improve health.

These theories haven't been substantiated by scientific evidence or through research studies. On the whole, the blood-type diet recommends eating healthy foods and avoiding artificial foods and highly processed and refined carbohydrates. But some of the food recommendations are challenging, to say the least.

Many of our clients have tried the program with limited success. A few find that it works for them really well, but this is a very small percentage.

> **Body of Knowledge**
>
> The blood-type diet recommends that people with type B blood eat lots of rabbit but not eat chicken. Try finding rabbit at a fast-food restaurant! Even lamb, recommended for those with type B and type AB blood, is darned hard to find when traveling or eating out with friends.

When you're on the blood-type diet, it's difficult to live a normal life, eat with your family, vacation, go on business trips, and eat in restaurants. When you consider some of the unusual foods that are recommended, you can easily see why. Depending on your blood type, you might be encouraged to eat such foods as rabbit, lamb, Ezekiel bread, and quinoa flour.

We don't have a problem with the overall concept or the eating recommendations themselves. We just can't imagine how a person could follow this program for a lifetime.

Food Combining Craziness

Food combining is an unusual concept for weight loss, although variations of this diet have been around since the 1930s. The premise is that certain foods don't digest well when you eat them with certain other foods. When you eat just the right foods in the right combinations, your weight will fall off.

In a nutshell, proteins shouldn't be eaten with starches, and fruits shouldn't be eaten with either proteins or starches. So a person could have meat and vegetables, or veggies and starches, or fruit all by itself. Not surprisingly, there's no scientific evidence to back up these digestion claims.

This diet system is sort of crazy. For instance, it recommends that you eat only fruits for the first 10 days and plenty of them. Obviously, this encourages you to overeat (that is, to eat beyond a 5 on the hunger scale). On day 11, you're told to eat a half-pound of bread, two tablespoons of butter, and three ears of corn. On day 19, you can have some complete protein. Obviously, the plan is unbalanced and will likely result in you missing essential nutrients, essential amino acids, and essential fatty acids.

This diet is a gimmick, is not in alignment with balanced nutrition, and can be dangerous to your health. It will cause your insulin levels to swing wildly and can put you into starvation metabolism, which causes fat storage and, ultimately, regaining any weight you've lost.

Please, forget food combining. Instead, eat as recommended in Part 3 of this book.

> **Thinspiration** _____
>
> The craziness of the food-combining diet should immediately raise a red flag that warns you to look elsewhere. Use your common sense when evaluating eating systems. Ask yourself, "Is this how my naturally thin friends eat?" Most people who are at their ideal size eat balanced, nutritious diets, and they definitely eat 0–5.

Eat as Paleo Man

To eat as the cavemen did is a simple concept: your diet should focus on the foods that our Paleolithic ancestors ate. Why? Because our bodies are basically the same as our primitive ancestors' bodies, so our diets should mirror theirs. The DNA of humans has changed less than 0.02 percent over the past 40,000 years. By contrast, grains (such as wheat and corn) were introduced into humankind's diet only about 10,000 years ago. In many parts of the world, some grains and other starches have only been added to the local diets in the past few thousand years.

In our opinion, by adopting the food intake of your ancient ancestors, you could improve your health and get to your ideal size.

One of the best-known primitive eating programs recommends that you eat lean meats, seafood, fish and eggs, plus plenty of fresh fruits and non-starchy vegetables. You eliminate all dairy, grains, legumes, sugar, and processed and artificial foods. The proportions of proteins, fats, and fruits and vegetables are close to what we recommend in Part 3.

You can eat as a caveman almost anywhere—at restaurants, at cocktail parties, and at a business lunch—although we suggest you use a few modern tools when you do, like a fork and knife instead of your fingers! The maintenance program is the same as the initial eating program, so the plan can work for your lifetime.

Weighty Warning

If a primitive eating program advocates eating as much as you want of permitted foods, don't take the advice. You should always tune in to your stomach's hunger signals to know when to eat and when to stop eating.

One important caution here: the plan is strict. Too strict, in our opinion. It leaves little room for a piece of pizza, a chocolate bar, or a scoop of ice cream. However, we feel that if you could eat the Paleo diet 80 percent of the time, you would be doing your size and health a favor.

You can use the basic insights of the Paleo Diet without becoming philosophically obsessed with it. Use common sense and don't make your treat foods into something bad or evil. Just eat them in moderation, as you would anything else. If the caveman had discovered chocolate 40,000 years ago, you can be sure he would have eaten some!

The Frequent-Eater Plans

These plans claim that the secret to weight loss lies in eating frequently. Most recommend about six small meals a day, usually a healthy mix of proteins, fats, and fruits and vegetables at every meal.

We like the balanced diet, but if you choose a frequent-eater plan, make sure that you only eat when you are hungry and stop when you are satisfied (that is, eat when you're at 0 and stop at or below a 5). If it's time for one of your small meals and you aren't hungry, wait until you are. There is no benefit in eating when you aren't hungry.

Some of the frequent-eater plans suggest you graze, which means you eat little bits of food all day long. Eating constantly works well for mammals such as cows and sheep, but it doesn't work the same way for humans. Your biology is not that of a ruminating animal. If it were, you also would have four stomachs and a cud. Just think of the exercise effort you would expend trying to keep all four tummies flat!

The Least You Need to Know

- Fasting for weight loss is usually ineffective and unhealthy.
- The more strict a vegetarian diet is, the more difficult it becomes to lose weight.
- Any food plan that is unbalanced or too difficult to maintain isn't going to work over the long term.
- If your food philosophy is making you fat or unhealthy, stop using it and make a change.

Chapter 24

Review of Diet Ideas

In This Chapter

- Weighing in: High protein versus low fat
- Examining mythological weight-burning foods
- Eating in the "Zone"
- Judging specialty diets

With so many diet books and programs available, how could you possibly choose? One says to avoid fat. The next one says to eat tons of lean protein. Another will tell you to eat lots of protein and fats but no carbohydrates. Yet another will tell you to eat in a "Zone." How can all of these approaches possibly work?

The answer is simple. On any given day, for some people, each of these diets work. We'll even bet that a few of them have worked for you … for a while. We're betting you're ready to get off the diet treadmill. Rather than having to choose your next diet and then the one after that, you want to settle at your ideal size and stay there for life. Let's see how some of these diet approaches stack up for long-term weight loss and health.

High-Protein Diets

Virtually everyone has tried some kind of high-protein diet. The most extreme plans encourage you to eat lots of meat, seafood, and fat and to avoid carbohydrates, even fruits and vegetables. In fact, the advocates of these eating plans want you to scrape the breading off your fish in a restaurant. You can eat as much meat and fat as you want provided you eat virtually no carbohydrates. Of course, you won't get fiber in your diet either.

Avoiding all carbohydrates, even vegetables and fruit, forces the body to find other sources of fuel, so the body will burn body fat for energy. So far, so good. But your body will also break down muscle protein to make glucose for energy. This is called glucogenesis. Your body uses muscle protein from all body muscles—the thighs, the arms, even the heart.

When your body burns fat while deprived of dietary carbohydrates, your body produces ketones. This activity is called *ketosis*. Ketosis does cause weight loss—mostly water weight. The high-protein diets that cause ketosis can be damaging to a person who already has liver or kidney problems.

> **Lean Lingo**
>
> **Ketosis** is a body state that occurs when you burn fat without enough glucose. This happens when your diet is low in carbohydrates. Ketosis is safe for most people, but not for persons whose health is already compromised.

With all this going on with high-protein, low-carbohydrate diets, is it any wonder that people tend to regain their weight quickly when the diet is over?

Is it worth it? Absolutely not. The high-protein diet taken to the extreme without any carbs is unhealthy. It lacks common sense. The high-protein diets recommend overeating, which always creates problems.

Low-Carb Diets

Most low-carb diet plans work very well. The books and programs recommend a balanced diet of meats, seafood, poultry, and eggs with plenty of vegetables and some fruit. They leave out the fluffy white starches, which no one needs—but many of us love.

Be sure you don't eat no-carb. That's asking for trouble because you'll be missing out on antioxidants, vitamins, minerals, and fiber. Continue to eat 5–10 servings of vegetables and fruit every day.

Don't be shy of eating fruit. You can have 2–3 servings a day, just don't eat all your servings at the same time. Since virtually all fruit is low-glycemic, most people won't have a problem with elevated blood sugar levels. If you have diabetes, learn which fruits work for you and how much.

We like low-carb eating plans because you can eat this way all of your life. And you can eat healthy low-carb fare in any restaurant—even in fast-food restaurants.

Low-Glycemic Diets

These eating programs are very similar to low-carb. You'll find almost identical food recommendations. The difference is how to count. With a low-carb diet, you'll count total carbs. With low-glycemic eating, you'll count total glycemic load.

You'll be eating animal proteins with fruits and vegetables. Any starches you eat will be rated low-glycemic, and you'll be able to eat limited amounts of these.

With low-glycemic eating, you keep your blood sugar levels and insulin levels in a safe range that prevents fat storage and encourages fat burning. The program is ideal for people with hypoglycemia and for those with diabetes. If you are metabolically resistant to weight loss, this is the plan for you.

Low-glycemic eating is very healthy, and you can stay on the eating plan for life. And, hurrah, the maintenance program is virtually identical to the diet program, so you won't need to make big changes to stay at your ideal size.

You can learn more about how to eat based on the glycemic index in the book, *The Complete Idiot's Guide to Glycemic Index Weight Loss*.

Weight-Burning Foods

Ahhh, those "magic" foods. If only weight loss were so simple. No single food will ever make your body burn enough fat to get you to your ideal size for life. Most will have no positive impact at all. So forget about relying on grapefruit, watermelon, or celery. The same with cabbage soup or any other specific food. All of these may be yummy foods to you, and they're terrific as part of a balanced eating plan, but they hold no magic.

Simple common sense should tell you that reliance on a particular food to get to your ideal size is doomed from the beginning. If you aren't eating a balanced diet, you aren't going to feel energized and healthy. There's a good chance your body will respond by going into starvation metabolism, and there's an even better chance you'll put back on any lost weight as soon as you come off the diet.

Forget about magic food theories. They're myths made popular by magazines trying to sell copies at the grocery store checkout.

> **Weighty Warning**
>
> You can help your body burn food more quickly in several ways, but grapefruit isn't one of them. No single food can do it. But you can inspire your body to burn food more quickly by increasing your metabolism through strength training and aerobic exercise, reducing stress, and avoiding starvation metabolism. An extra caution about grapefruit: grapefruit juice can interfere with certain prescription medications such as statins, which are cholesterol-lowering medications, beta-blockers, and calcium channel blockers.

Low-Fat Diets

Is fat the enemy? Many low-fat diets recommend that you reduce fat to 10 percent or less of your total caloric intake to make your heart healthier. This isn't enough fat for you to lose weight and have good health. The low-fat diets either don't recommend or ignore altogether the essential fatty acids that assist with weight loss and improve heart health. They advocate eating low-fat processed foods that are filled with sugars and high-glycemic starches. Recent studies show that eating high-glycemic starches, such as French bread, bagels, and cookies, will increase your LDL (low-density lipoproteins, the bad cholesterol) levels. Extremely low-fat diets are not a good path to life-long thinness.

Yes, it is important to eat less dietary fat. However, avoid relying on an extreme low-fat eating plan. Its recommendations are not nutritionally sound and can be harmful. You can have a healthy heart without excessive restrictions on your eating.

Many low-fat diets fail to recommend consuming essential fatty acids, and many promote eating high-glycemic carbohydrates. You need essential fatty acids to keep your heart healthy, and the high-glycemic starches raise LDL cholesterol levels, contributing to heart disease.

An ideal and healthy range for eating fat in your diet is to eat between 25 and 30 percent of your calories from fat. The American Heart Association recommends 30 percent. Yet many Americans eat upward of 50 percent of their daily calories as fat. So if this is you, you and your heart will benefit from cutting your fat intake; eat a moderately low-fat diet.

Zone Eating

The basic premise of the "Zone" eating program is to eat about 40 percent carbohydrates, 30 percent protein, and 30 percent fat on a daily basis. This is excellent. So far, so good. But there's no reason why you will lose weight eating this way unless you also only eat when hungry and stop before you're full.

Among the food recommendations, some foods, such as eggs, are tagged as bad for you. We don't agree with this.

Eating the specific nutrient ratios, give or take, can be done over a lifetime.

Packaged foods for zone eating are now available. The ingredients are healthful, and we love that the foods don't need to be frozen or refrigerated, so they could be convenient for traveling. Remember to use packaged foods as a convenience item, eating them once in a while but not every day. Packaged foods do not contain your daily five fresh fruits and vegetables, so be sure to eat them in addition to a prepackaged convenience meal.

Overall, Zone eating is fine. Make sure that you also eat 0–5 to lose weight.

The No-Sugar Way

These diets recommend that a person avoid high-glycemic starches and sugars and instead limit carbohydrate intake to fruits and vegetables. Believers cite studies showing that high-glycemic carbohydrates stimulate the body to overproduce insulin, thus prompting fat storage. Usually these diets offer balanced eating, with a recommendation of 30 percent proteins, 30 percent fats, and 40 percent carbohydrates. So far, we agree that this is a good and healthy way of eating.

But then some of the no-sugar diets get off track. Some recommend aspartame, sucralose, or saccharine as sugar substitutes. Please don't use these at all. Some no-sugar plans recommend food combining, which you can totally ignore. Some of the plans suggest that you are allowed one day or one meal a week to eat anything you want. We abhor this idea. A binge day is not healthy or good common sense. In fact, it encourages a person to overeat and thus harm his or her body.

Weighty Warning

Beware of any diet systems that highly recommend that you eat artificial foods such as artificial sweeteners, preservatives, and colorings. Growing evidence suggests that these are harmful to your health.

Although we support the premise of reducing sugars and starches, we don't like the rigidity and strict rules. Maintenance is difficult when the rules don't allow for eating a piece of wedding cake or a burrito. If you relax the rules to allow yourself to eat some high-glycemic starches as a condiment and you stay away from artificial sweeteners, you could find that these programs work for a lifetime.

Diet in a Box

Many diet systems offer packaged foods that are available in the grocery store, discount stores, and on the Internet. The same criteria apply to these foods as to any others. Read the labels.

♦ Do they contain artificial ingredients?

♦ Are they low-fat?

♦ Do they want you to substitute soy protein for meat, poultry, and fish?

♦ Are they full of sodium and salt?

♦ Do they contain high-glycemic carbohydrates?

If the answer to any of these questions is "yes," consider other alternatives. Just buy regular food and eat 0–5.

The Least You Need to Know

♦ High-protein, low-carbohydrate diet plans can work short-term, but without plenty of fresh fruits and vegetables, these plans fall short of good nutrition.

♦ Because your body needs fat (especially essential fatty acids) to release fat stores, eating an extremely low-fat diet can inhibit weight loss.

♦ Specialty eating plans as a whole are seldom nutritionally balanced and might not deliver lifelong weight management.

♦ What works for long-term, lifelong weight loss is *you* and not any special system.

Chapter 25

Medical and Counseling Approaches to Weight Loss

In This Chapter

◆ Counseling for weight loss

◆ Risks and rewards of weight-loss drugs

◆ Liposuction and tummy tucks

◆ Stomach surgery to control eating

Hasn't everyone who is overweight wished for the perfect little pill? The one that would melt away the fat virtually overnight? Of course. Has there ever been one? Yes and no.

The medical profession and pharmaceutical companies have been searching for "fat fixes" for many years. They know that solving our overeating problems with a pill would help lots of us improve our health, make us happier …, and make *them* a lot of money. They keep trying.

Or maybe doctors can just make our stomachs smaller so that we have less urge to eat. Actually, they can.

Let's take a closer look at how the medical profession and the counseling professions are tackling the weight problem.

One-on-One Coaching

If you're at your wits' end and don't know where to turn or what to do to get the weight off, consider using a weight-loss coach, a psychiatrist, psychologist, or registered dietitian. He or she can help you make sense of your weight-loss issues and can help you determine what will work best for you.

A weight-loss counseling professional can give you helpful insights into the root emotional cause of your overeating and can suggest a plan for healing your inner overeating self. Plus, some can actually recommend a doable food and eating plan, a practical exercise plan, an accountability system, emotional support, a feedback system so you can make changes if the program needs adjusting, and suggestions for supplementation. When interviewing weight-loss counseling professionals, you should select an individual who is already at his or her ideal size and has appropriate credentials or a great track record.

> **Body of Knowledge**
>
> Weight-loss counseling professionals are not all the same. For instance, one might emphasize detailed eating plans but might not give you tips to tackle the emotional issues surrounding your weight. Another might help you with a broader approach to weight loss by redirecting your eating habits. Investigate your "coach" before selecting. Check out references and referrals.

To ensure your success, be sure to tell all. Yes, even about the two drinks you have every evening or how quickly you get to the bottom of ice cream cartons. Francie was a sweet single woman who kept trying to lose some stubborn weight. One day, she calmly confessed that maybe, just maybe, the munchies she got from smoking pot every night before bed might be part of her problem!

Yes, your coach needs to know everything that's relevant. If you can't divulge your little eating secrets, don't waste your time and money.

Hypnosis

We give hypnosis mixed reviews. It works well for some people and not for others. Weight loss is not easily tackled by hypnosis. The problem is the nature of eating. Because we all need to eat, the hypnotist can't use an all-or-nothing approach, which works well for phobias and for smoking cessation.

If you want to try hypnosis, keep an open mind. It could work!!! As with any professional service, check out the hypnotist's credentials and check their references.

The Search for the Perfect Pill

In the 1950s, there were amphetamines. Diet pills. Speed. They worked pretty well. They hyped a person up enough to burn calories. Eventually, we learned that they also ruined a person's health. They were highly addictive. They weren't safe. The FDA pulled them off the market.

Then, in the 1990s, another diet pill was formulated that produced great results for many people. Fen-phen soothed its users, and they no longer wanted to overeat. They lost weight almost effortlessly. Unfortunately, within a couple of years, several of them were dead. Fen-phen silently was causing pulmonary hypertension leading to lung and heart damage. This combination of pills wasn't safe. The FDA pulled them off the market.

The search for the perfect prescription diet pill by the major drug companies goes on. Weight loss is big business, and we're all eager for the pharmaceutical industry to find a successful and healthy weight-loss pill.

Researchers are now exploring genetic coding and are actually looking for a way to alter a person's biology to prevent the body from storing fat.

> **Weighty Warning**
>
> All prescription drugs for weight loss bring with them serious side effects. Make sure that you are well informed before you make your decision. Also, be sure to learn the average weight loss of users and how quickly users regain their weight when they stop taking the drug.

Even though obesity and being overweight have been declared a health epidemic, these conditions aren't caused by a bacteria or virus like other epidemics. Our collective chubbiness is usually caused by a lack of regular exercise, overeating, and poor food choices. Some other important causes are food allergies, toxin build-up, high insulin levels, and some medications. Here is information on some of the current drugs used for weight loss. They are only recommended for people who are obese, meaning they have a BMI equal to or greater than 30. If you are considering a weight-loss drug, keep these two questions in mind:

- What are the side effects, and can I live with them?

- What are the chances I will regain my weight?

Here's what is available by prescription.

Meridia

This pharmaceutical is also known as Reducil, and the common name is sibutramine. It is an appetite suppressant that is intended to be used with a low-calorie diet and exercise program. It stimulates various appetite-control centers in the brain and affects levels of brain neurotransmitters, which also can reduce appetite. It costs about $85 a month and is seldom covered by insurance. (Costs can vary considerably.)

> **Body of Knowledge**
>
> All weight-loss drugs come with recommendations that include using a low-calorie diet and an exercise program. Even with medication, a person still needs to limit food intake and exercise regularly. Keep that in mind if you are considering using medications for weight loss.

Sibutramine has been deemed safe for only one year of use. You can expect to keep your weight off for up to a year. It's only recommended for people with a BMI of 30 or higher or for those with a BMI higher than 27 who are at risk for diabetes, high blood pressure, or high cholesterol.

Unwanted side effects can include raised heart rates and higher blood pressure. Sales of Reducil have been suspended in Italy after 50 reports of adverse reactions and 2 deaths. Overall, reports suggest that 34 deaths have been associated with taking this drug.

Acomplia

This drug, developed in France, is also called "rimonabant." It works by blocking a pleasure center in the brain, which helps people eat less, while acting directly on fat cells to prevent weight gain. The drug is not yet available in the United States.

Test results are positive. 3,040 obese people in the test group each lost an average of 19 pounds over two years while taking Acomplia. Those who took a placebo lost an average of 5.5 pounds.

Other positive results showed a reduction in the number of people who had metabolic syndrome. Many people kept the weight off for more than two years.

Side effects include nausea, dizziness, and diarrhea. Some people—2.8 percent—dropped out of the study because of depression.

The people in the study didn't lose large amounts of weight, and even with losing 19 pounds, many were still obese after two years. This medication could be valuable, but don't expect to fit into your size 8 jeans if you're starting out in the obese category.

Xenical

Also called "Orlistat," this drug is used for the treatment of chronic obesity. It reduces your body's ability to absorb fat from the foods you eat. In essence, it is a fat blocker. It works best if you are able to stick to a low-calorie diet and a regular exercise regime.

The side effects include gas, increased frequency of bowel movements, and fatty/oily stool. We have heard of people who "leak" (experience fecal incontinence) while on this drug.

Since your body needs fat, especially essential fatty acids, we hate to think that users miss the benefits from the fats they eat. Bottom line, this drug is unpleasant. Clinical trials show it's safe for up to two years of use.

Phentermine

This half of the banned fen-phen weight-loss pill is still approved for use. Also called "Adipex," Phentermine is an appetite suppressant that is similar in molecular structure to amphetamines. It is habit-forming. Phentermine increases your heart rate and blood pressure and decreases your appetite. Because it is chemically similar to amphetamines, a person could become addicted to this drug.

Needless to say, a person can't stay on phentermine for a lifetime. The likelihood of regaining your weight when you stop taking this drug is extremely high.

Other Drug Possibilities

Some medications that have been approved by the FDA for other medical conditions are now being considered for use as weight-loss drugs. The following show promise:

◆ Wellbutrin is an antidepressant. People using it might experience small weight loss.

◆ Topamax is an antiepilepsy drug. It has been shown to suppress appetite but can have serious side effects.

Fat Removal ... Literally

Perhaps you have thought that rather than trim the amount of food you eat, you could just pay a surgeon to trim the fat out of your body. We're talking about liposuction, tummy tucks, and other surgical fat-removal techniques.

Liposuction and tummy tucks certainly can take away the fat. The surgeon cuts it out or siphons it out. When you come out of surgery, you will have thinner thighs, a smaller derriere, or a flatter tummy. These days, plastic surgery isn't just limited to below the waist. People are having their upper arms, waists, breasts, and other body places liposuctioned.

If you've inherited saddlebags that no amount of exercise or diet will reduce, liposuction could be a choice. But we need to tell you that those saddlebags can grow back even after liposuction. Body fat tends to be stored in the same places as before surgery. Several girlfriends have had their thighs "done" more than once.

Is liposuction or a tummy tuck for you? Only you and your bank account know the answer to that question. They're definitely *not* long-term answers to your weight problems. A surgeon can't cut out your poor eating habits. The weight will come right back if you overeat. So approach surgery knowing that your long-term success depends on eating as a thin person for the rest of your life.

Lean Lingo

Liposuction is a surgical process in which fat is suctioned from the areas of your body where excess amounts are stored. A plastic surgeon will make one or more small incisions through your skin layers and then suction out the fat cells. The procedure is usually performed in a doctor's office or clinic rather than a hospital.

Liposuction is serious surgery. It requires anesthetics and can have complications. Make sure that you find a surgeon who is board-certified and get recommendations from your regular doctor. Good plastic surgeons want you to be at your ideal weight *before* they operate so that they can take away the saddlebags you were, in essence, born with.

Plastic surgery is expensive and is not covered by health insurance. Expect to pay several thousand dollars for a surgeon to rid you of saddlebags or give you a flat tummy.

Stomach Surgery

This is serious stuff. Don't even think of this drastic step unless you have a BMI of 40 or above. The operation, commonly referred to as "stomach stapling," is called "gastric bypass" or *bariatric* surgery. More than 146,301 bariatric surgeries were performed in the United States in 2003. This number is growing yearly. Many people have good results—they lose weight and keep it off. The physical surgery is only the first phase of the weight-loss process. The next phase is the one that lasts for years—eating frequent small meals that are nutrient-dense. This phase requires major behavioral modification and discipline.

The surgery is not a guarantee that you won't regain your weight. We have participants in our weight-loss classes who have had their stomachs stapled. Some of them are still paying off the loans for their surgery, yet they're back in class to lose weight. The surgery works when you change your eating habits for life. To do this, take classes in how to eat and cook differently and attend support group meetings or counseling to ensure your long-term success.

> **Lean Lingo**
>
> **Bariatric** surgery is derived from the Greek words for weight and treatment. Bariatric surgery is a major operation that (a) seals off most of the stomach to reduce the amount of food one can eat, and (b) rearranges the small intestine to reduce the calories the body can absorb.

The Roux-en-Y is abdominal surgery in which the stomach is stapled to a lower area in the small intestine—bypassing approximately 155 centimeters of small intestine. Problems with this surgery include increased complications of leaking at the bypass sites, significant and persistent diarrhea, and a mortality rate of about 1.5 percent. About 20 percent of patients need additional surgery to remedy complications and 30 percent develop nutritional deficiencies.

The adjustable gastric band is a new and reportedly safer and easier form of stomach surgery. The adjustable gastric band (or the abdominal band, as it is sometimes called) has been more popular in Europe, although it is now being used in the United States. It is safer then Roux-en-y surgery, which until now has been more commonly used in the United States. People lose two to three pounds per week over the first year and then usually maintain weight after that.

The adjustable gastric band is installed laparoscopically through small incisions in the abdomen rather than through a major incision. Essentially, the band clamps around the stomach to limit the amount of food you can get into it. A valve is inserted in the chest area, and the doctor can use it to tighten or loosen the band.

If you choose bypass surgery, here's what you need to know:

◆ It's not a quick fix or a "walk in the park." This drastic alternative includes pain, hospitalization, and high risk factors.

◆ You must change your eating habits after the surgery and keep them for life. Absolutely no more overeating.

◆ You might or might not lose all the weight you want to lose. On average, a person loses 60 percent of their excess weight. So if you're 100 pounds overweight, you could expect to lose 60 pounds.

◆ You must be 100 pounds overweight with a BMI of 40+ to qualify.

◆ Insurance seldom pays for bariatric surgery.

◆ You are at risk for nutritional deficiencies, so you'll need to take vitamin and mineral supplements.

◆ Seldom is bariatric surgery recommended for teenagers or people over 60.

Even after stomach surgery, you must make a lifetime commitment to exercise and diet to stay at your ideal size. Because this is really serious surgery, be prepared to handle complications and side issues. Some people find the surgery to be a dream come true. They have much less appetite and few side effects. Others have trouble eating even simple foods and risk an increased problem of vomiting after meals. No one can predict your outcome. Before you downsize your stomach, learn everything you can about the process and talk to others who have had the surgery. Many good Internet sites offer chat rooms for you to meet people who have had the surgery.

Although there are exceptions, don't expect this surgery to be covered by your health insurance.

The Least You Need to Know

◆ Prescription drugs for weight loss have a track record of serious side effects and seldom solve lifetime weight-loss issues.

◆ Consider using diet pills only if your BMI is 30 or above and you and your doctor agree that you must lose weight for health reasons.

◆ Cosmetic surgery, such as liposuction, is not intended for weight loss but rather to reshape the body.

◆ Bariatric or gastric bypass surgery is major surgery that can have serious complications; it should be considered only by the seriously obese whose BMI is 40 or above.

Part 7

Get Your Mind-Set Right

As you lose weight, you will emerge from your fat "skin" with your body transformed into your ideal size. In this part of the book, we show you how to greet the world as a thin person. By adopting the mindset of being thin, you'll say good-bye forever to your fat self. You'll part ways with your fat thoughts, emotions, and behaviors. You'll order from restaurant menus with confidence and enjoy celebrations and parties with grace and ease. And you'll surround yourself with a support group to help you solidify your progress.

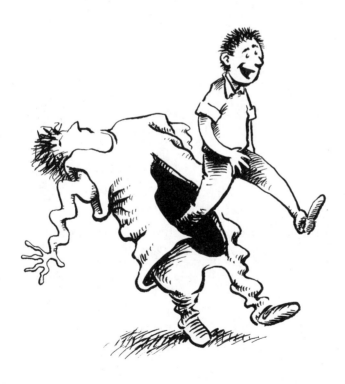

26

Think Yourself Thin

In This Chapter

- ◆ Using mental power
- ◆ Having clear intentions
- ◆ Being in charge
- ◆ Dealing with naysayers

Can you get to your ideal size by just thinking so? Yes, you can. We know people who have done it. You can give up having a weight issue. Just walk away from it. Adopt the attitude of "been there, done that." Convince yourself that you are already at your ideal size. How can you do this? By using your mental and emotional resources to make it so. Notice that we didn't say to use willpower and self-discipline. By now you have enough experience with weight loss to know these don't work, so let's take a different approach. We suspect it is one you haven't tried before.

Believing Is Seeing

Never underestimate the power of your mental outlook. Researchers tell us that the brain doesn't distinguish between what you imagine and what is real. Yes, if you imagine that you are at your ideal size, your subconscious doesn't know whether it is fact or fiction. The more you imagine and the more you turn away conflicting thoughts, the closer you get to being effortlessly thin.

People who are naturally thin do not think they are fat. They don't worry about what to eat, when to diet, or how to diet. The thoughts wouldn't cross their minds. Do the same for yourself. Here's how.

Cut Excuses Out of Your Thought Menu

You and only you are totally responsible for the size of your body. It wasn't the advertising that put the food into your mouth. It wasn't anyone else, either. It was only one thing—you. We want you to stop using excuses and take full responsibility for the size of your body. This action empowers you to make the changes necessary to get to your ideal size.

> ### Body of Knowledge
>
> The research on the power of thoughts overwhelmingly supports getting your thinking in alignment with being thin for life. Get rid of any fat thinking and behaviors. If using the power of thoughts works for Olympic athletes and professional ballplayers, it can work for you.

> ### Thinspiration
>
> Learning to eat as if you were already thin can be fun. Take your thin friends out to lunch or dinner and observe how they eat. Then model their healthy eating behaviors, such as being picky eaters and not cleaning their plates.

Yes, we mean that mom, the kids, the spouse, the hormones, and on and on are not the real reason you have a weight issue. It was solely how you reacted to your life situations. For example, when Lucy got over the fact that her son had learning disabilities and that she had to deal with the situation rather than eat over it, she was finally able to release the fat. We know this sounds really tough and a bit ruthless, but we also know you want to be your ideal size.

You are in charge. Act in charge of your eating. Be picky and be impolite. After all, it is your body and not anyone else's. You have our permission to be obnoxious if necessary to avoid eating what you don't want or need.

If you find yourself wanting to make excuses for your size, stop mid-word (just like you should stop mid-bite if you were done eating). Then take it back, rephrase it, and say it in such a way that you are responsible and in charge. For example, if you say or even think, "I feel fat today," reword it and instead say aloud, "I feel thin today." Turning around your thoughts like this gives you power.

Forgiveness as Weight-Loss Aid

Perhaps you started gaining weight from the stress of a major—or even minor—life event. Such things as divorce or loss of a loved one can trigger overeating for consolation. So can getting older and feeling older.

If you can release the trauma and sadness from such events and the people associated with them, you can often come to terms with overeating. To do this, use the power of forgiveness. *Forgiveness* is the act of pardoning without harboring grievances. The key to success with forgiveness is persistence, tenacity, and desire.

In virtually every religion in the world, forgiveness is considered to be a highly sacred and spiritual practice. We agree. We also know that forgiveness has great power to heal wounds and release weight. So, if you feel burdened by past life events, as if you are still carrying around their weight, use forgivenesses. Here's how:

First make a list of everyone who was involved in your weight issue. Be sure to include yourself. Then make up some forgivenesses and write them down. Use the formula, "I, (*fill in your name*), forgive you for (*whatever the issue*)." Also write forgivenesses for yourself, such as, "I, (*fill in your name*), forgive myself for (*whatever the issue*)."

For yourself, you could write the following:

> I forgive myself for overeating.
> I forgive myself for getting older.
> I forgive myself for being overweight.
> I forgive myself for abusing my body with too much food.
> I forgive myself for not exercising.

One client came back to class the next week having begun the forgiveness homework exercise. She told the class that she had written 27 pages of forgivenesses, and she still wasn't finished forgiving her mother. But she said it was really a great feeling.

Although it might sound somewhat shallow to forgive a person so that you can lose weight, well, if you haven't forgiven them already, perhaps it's time. And your weight situation presents a treasured opportunity to let go of past grievances.

We figure it doesn't matter why you forgive. It just matters that you do.

Tell the Truth

Tell the real truth to yourself with compassion about what you eat, how much you eat, when you eat, and if you ate above a 5 or started eating above 0. We have clients who fudge when they record their hunger numbers. Now, just who are they cheating and why? Are they trying to look good to themselves?

We suggest that you use the form that follows to record your hunger numbers and food intake every day, for every meal, every snack, and every nibble. Record everything you put into your mouth except water. Be ruthlessly honest with yourself. That way, you get excellent results. You get the results you want.

Date:

Time	Beginning Hunger #	Item	Amount	Ending Hunger #	Time
_____	_____	_____	_____	_____	_____
_____	_____	_____	_____	_____	_____

Percentage of day I was a thin person in mind and behavior = _____ %

So typical meals look this way:

Date: 02/02/05

Time	Beginning Hunger #	Item	Amount	Ending Hunger #	Time
8:35 A.M.	0	salmon green apple	card deck size small	5	9:05 A.M.
6:15 P.M.	0	roast beef spinach salad brownie	card deck size bowl small	5	7:00 P.M.

Percentage of day I was a thin person in mind and behavior = 100%

Notice that you don't need to weigh and measure your food. We aren't asking you to weigh and measure your body, and we certainly aren't going to ask you to weigh and measure your food. Just record what you ate. You know whether it's too much food.

Record your food intake and hunger numbers every day until you are comfortably at your ideal size. You can continue as long as you want. If your jeans ever get tight, record your food intake and hunger numbers until they fit comfortably. We have done this off and on for more than 20 years. You'll find it a great maintenance plan.

Ban Diet Paraphernalia

People who have the mindset of being thin do not keep diet stuff around the house. Let's say that you didn't own a dog, never owned a dog, and didn't have any plans to have a dog. Yet you owned a dog dish, a leash, dog food, and purchased books on raising and breeding dogs. You would appear nuts.

Ditto believing you are thin. Thin people don't have kitchens stocked full of diet and low-cal foods. They don't have large clothes in their closets just in case they regain their weight. All the clothes in their closets fit. They get rid of clothes because they are worn out, soiled, or out of style, not because they don't fit. They don't own dozens of books on weight-loss plans. If they did, they would seem nutty.

Toss out your cache of diet paraphernalia. Give it away. Get it out of your sight. It will mess up your thin thinking to constantly see a food scale on the kitchen counter. Be consistent inside and out with being a thin person.

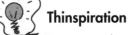 **Thinspiration**

Toss out anything in your refrigerator that you purchased with the hope that it would make you thinner. Get rid of low-fat salad dressings, low-fat ice cream and yogurt. Remember to get rid of fake butter and those "spreads" that are filled with transfatty acids that are designed to taste like the real thing. And what about that low-fat cheese? Now go to the grocery store and buy real foods just like naturally thin people eat.

Ban Fat Thoughts

Stop telling yourself you are fat. Stop saying you are so big that .... Refuse to believe it even when the mirror says otherwise. You could be your own worst enemy when it comes to weight.

When Linda was overweight, she cried about it a lot and constantly talked about her problems with her weight, eating, and food. One day, as her husband was once again drying her tears, he said, "I think things would get a whole lot better if you would just stop telling yourself you're fat."

Thinspiration _____

Take one day and monitor your thoughts about your weight, eating, and size. You might be amazed at the sheer number of negative messages you send to yourself. These kinds of thoughts only reinforce your weight issue and make it more difficult to attain your ideal size.

Linda, already wounded, said, "So what do you know?" Later she had to apologize when she realized he knew a whole lot.

She stopped crying about her weight issue.
She stopped talking about it.
She stopped commiserating with her fat friends.
She stopped buying diet foods.
She stopped telling herself she was fat—and ugly.
She stopped seeing food as the enemy.

She gained control of her eating and lost weight down to her ideal size.

How High Is Your Desire?

Ask yourself what percentage of the time you are willing to think and act as a thin person. How often are you willing to eat 0 to 5? How often will you eat sensuously and beautifully?

If your answer is about 50 percent of the time, your odds of success are less than 50 percent, more like about 5 percent. However, if you can give it your all, or 100 percent, for as long as it takes, you will definitely get to your ideal size.

But "as long as it takes" is sort of meaningless to schedule in your daily planner. So instead, ask yourself this question every day: "What percentage of my day was I a full participant in being a thin person?" If you had moments that were less than 100 percent, review each situation and ask yourself what you could have done better.

As long as you know deep in your heart that you are thinking and eating as a thin person every day, you absolutely know you will reach your goal.

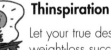

Thinspiration _____

Let your true desire fuel your weight-loss success. Wanting may not be the same as getting, but without the wanting, you most likely won't get. Build your desire and pave the way to your inner and outer success.

When Suzie arrived at a luncheon date with a college friend with her hunger number way below 0, she could have eaten the proverbial horse, so to speak. Suzie dove into the white bread and then proceeded to eat all of her lasagna and salad. When she stood up to leave, she was between a 9 and a 10 on the hunger scale. Looking back on her experience, she could have ordered a glass of fruit juice when the waiter first came to the table and then sipped it slowly until her hunger level rose to 0. Then, when the entrée came, she would have had the ability to eat normally—that is, to eat from 0–5.

At the end of each day, ask yourself what percentage of the day you ate and thought as a thin person.

The Naysayers

You've met naysayers before. These people tell you it will never work, that they have tried that method before and it didn't work for them, so why should it work for you?

Beware the naysayers who notice that you are eating differently and try to break your resolve. Others will lecture you on how weight loss really works and will let you know that you are doing it all wrong. Some actually push food on you and insist you eat what they want you to eat.

Maria was obviously overweight and was enjoying an ice cream cone while sitting outside on a bench at a popular neighborhood shopping area. A strange woman approached her, sat down next to her, and said, "Are you sure you should be eating that ice cream cone?" Then she proceeded to tell Maria that she had lost all sorts of weight recently and told her how she did it. Maria just got up and walked away. The nerve of some people. We would like to think that this strange woman had good intentions—but she sure didn't have good boundaries.

How do you handle these people, whether they are doing it for your own best good or not? First and foremost, don't tell just anyone you're on a weight-loss program. Even if people ask, you don't need to tell them everything. If they notice you have lost weight and want to know how, refer them to this book. It's best to avoid a long story with detailed descriptions. Here are some suggestions for handling these pushy people:

- **The food pusher.** Say one of these two things: "Oh, no thanks, not right now, it looks delicious, but I'm saving room for dinner." Or say, "I'm just not hungry right now. It looks delicious, perhaps later."

- **The family member food pusher who wants you to eat more dessert or go back for seconds.** Put your hand across your tummy and say, "Thanks, your food was wonderful, but I just can't fit in another bite."

- **The "Are you sure you should be eating that?" person.** Answer "Absolutely!" and walk away.

Thinspiration

Build yourself a base of good support. First create the support within yourself and then find support in books, friends, and the Internet. Use this support when anyone challenges your goals and your weight-loss program.

- **The know-it-all-about-dieting person.** Say thanks but no thanks, especially if they aren't at their ideal size. It is best to learn from someone who has already mastered weight, not someone who is still trying to figure it out.

- **The fat friend.** This one is tough because it is possible you could lose some fat friends along the way if you master your weight. To stay friends, find other mutual interests.

- **Any potential naysayer.** The less you say, the less they can hurt you.

If you do happen to get in the path of a naysayer, as soon as you escape, be sure to repeat your inner mantra—see the following section—to yourself until any inner turmoil goes away and you get recentered as a thin person.

The Inner Mantra

Directing your thoughts to being thin is really hard. After all, you have years of scripts and self-talk that do anything but affirm your thin self. That's why we recommend you use the ideal size *affirmation*. This is the only one you need to use.

It goes like this, "I, (*insert first name*), am now a healthy and thin person. I wear a size (*insert desired size*), and I do what healthy and thin people do."

This statement affirms exactly what you want. If the word "thin" for you doesn't mean what it means to us, change it so that you are comfortable. Most often a person will change it to "lean." But we urge you not to change anything else. For example, don't change it to say, "I deserve to be thin." That is a lame and actually ineffective affirmation. Our response would be, "So what if you deserve to be thin? Deserving and being are two different things."

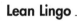

Lean Lingo

An **affirmation** is a carefully written positive statement declaring that you already have what you want. It usually starts with the words "I am" and states in present tense your desire as if you already have it.

The secret of this affirmation is that it declares you are already there. Yes, you will be shaking things up in your mind. This is good. You will be creating cognitive dissonance in your mind. Since this makes you uncomfortable, your insides will work hard to bring about compliance with your affirmation. Getting to your ideal size will require less and less thought and effort. In fact, you will be amazed at how easy it is to eat 0–5 after a couple months of using the affirmation.

To use the affirmation, say it aloud at least three times in a row three times a day. Yes, you can say it in private. That's a great start. It works even more quickly if you write it. That's right, write the affirmation 10 times every day. Purchase a spiral notebook or a journal and write the affirmation 10 times every day. Do it with meaning and care. At first, parts of your psyche will rebel. Let them. The writing will, over time, convince them that you are indeed a healthy and thin person.

If a situation comes up that challenges you, such as the desire to stress eat or if your favorite donuts show up at work and you aren't at 0, say your affirmation to yourself. Save the donut until you are once again at a 0.

Lucy continued to write her weight-loss affirmation for six months after she had reached her ideal size. She has stayed at her ideal size for more than 20 years. The time spent was a terrific investment.

Affirmations are one of the strongest and most effective tools for achieving your ideal size. We know plenty of people for whom this has worked. We also know people who have met their life's soul mate, improved their vision, and found terrific jobs by using the power of affirmations.

In a sense, you already affirm every day all day long. You have been affirming that you have an overweight body for years. Now change the "CD" and get what you really want.

What Is Your Intention?

Getting to your ideal size once and for all changes your life in many ways. Make sure that you are ready to live with the changes. They can be wonderful, and yet even wonderful changes can be unsettling and might take some time to get used to. To aid you in making those changes, you can use the following intention statements. These are very powerful and can let you make major changes in your weight and your life.

◆ I am now a size _____ in body, mind, and spirit.

   Getting to your ideal size just in your body without mental and spiritual alignment can make you gain your weight back really fast. When all aspects of you are totally aligned with being and with staying at your ideal size, you will.

◆ I am happy, comfortable, and safe being at my ideal size.

For many people, feeling happy, comfortable, and safe at a smaller size can seem impossible. They have built a fortress with their body for protection. Find real ways that you can be happy, comfortable, and safe and not use your body as a fortress.

♦ I honor my body and its messages.

This refers to all the body's messages: the need to eat, the need to stop eating, and the needs for sleep, relaxation, exercise, and movement. You may have been taught to ignore the body's signals as an indication of inner strength. Now it's time to learn that a person can't be a good caretaker of the body by ignoring it.

♦ I love, enjoy, and appreciate my body.

Perhaps as you were growing up, you were taught that the body is bad. However, we figure that the body is how you get through this life. Without a body, well, you wouldn't be here. We find that when people can love, enjoy, and appreciate their bodies, often overeating as a subtle form of self abuse ends. Most of our weight-loss clients are "body" people. They require lots of physical activity— either passive or active—to feel good, to be creative, and to be happy.

♦ I honor all of my emotions and use them responsibly.

Rather than stuffing emotions with food, which is not using emotions responsibly, learn how to use and express them with love. Also, remember to lift your moods with cardio/aerobic exercise to get the endorphin lift.

♦ I am in harmony with being at my ideal size.

Be sure that all of the aspects of you can function fully and excellently when you are at your ideal size. If you have a tiny voice inside that is fearful or even alarmed at the thought, talk with that part until you understand the fear and can make changes so that all of you is in harmony.

♦ I honor my sexual energy and express it appropriately.

Sexual energy as we use it here is a fabulous life-force power that can be used to enhance all of your life. It is not only about physical intimacy but rather sexual energy in all its forms. Even if you do not have a spouse or lover, you are still expressing sexual energy in how you work, walk, talk, and eat. No, we're not in any way talking about promiscuity. We are talking about being in the flow of joy, abundance, and love.

To start using these intentions, set aside some time. Then take each one in turn and say the intention to yourself. As resistance comes up, listen to your inner resistant reasons and then repeat the intention to yourself. Do this over and over again until you can feel in harmony or in congruence with each intention.

These intentions were carefully designed to include the biggest fears and resistances a person has about being at his or her ideal size. At the class session a week after we give these intentions as homework, the participants return looking radiant, as if years of weight gain have been lifted from their bodies (and for some of them, a dress size has been lifted also).

Thinspiration

Make these new ways of thinking a part of your daily life. Think about them, or say them to yourself during idle moments, such as when waiting for the elevator, waiting at a traffic light, or standing in line at the grocery store. You can't overdo them and repetition brings the rewards you desire.

Using the power of your mind and doing some mental and spiritual work can magnify your weight-loss efforts. The mental and spiritual work is like a booster engine, accelerating your weight-loss progress and lightening up your life.

The Least You Need to Know

♦ Accessing the power of your mind through affirmations can greatly accelerate your weight-loss progress.

♦ When you totally own your weight issues as your own and take full responsibility for your eating by giving up excuses, you can make consistent progress.

♦ Use forgiveness to get beyond any emotional and spiritual barriers to being your ideal size.

♦ Use intentions to clear out any fears about being your ideal size and use them to steer your mind toward reaching your goal.

Chapter **27**

Eat Out Fearlessly

In This Chapter

- Eating out with confidence
- Knowing what to order
- Sharing meals, bringing home leftovers
- Finding a healthy choice in every cuisine

Imagine eating out at any kind of restaurant—fast food, gourmet dining, or an all-you-can-eat buffet—without thinking about losing weight. Thin people don't think about dieting when they eat out. Why should you? Instead, eat like you're already at your ideal size!

Does this mean you can pig out? Of course not. When you're enjoying life at your ideal size, why would you ever pig out? It doesn't make sense.

So how do you eat out like someone at his or her ideal size? Actually, it's not hard. Every dining-out opportunity can help you reach and stay at your ideal size, even as you thoroughly enjoy the tastes and pleasures of the food. In this chapter, we tell you how.

What Eating Out Is About

Twenty-five years ago, forecasters predicted that Americans would begin to eat out much more often. Were they ever right! Why do we do it? For starters, eating out is convenient. Our lives seem busier than ever before,

Lean Lingo

To **dine** means to eat beautifully. Dining means thinking about your hunger number, giving thanks for your food, eating slowly, having a good time, and stopping eating when your stomach is comfortable. You can dine any time you eat out, even at fast-food restaurants. You can also, of course, dine at home.

and we prefer not to take time to purchase and prepare foods. Second, we like to be served. It's just plain nice to have someone else prepare and serve food to us. Finally, it's for pleasure. We eat out for new tastes, for superb dishes, for relaxation, as a treat, to get away from the house, and for all sorts of pleasurable reasons.

Plain old nourishment is the least important reason. This is a good thing, actually. When you're eating out, you want the camaraderie, the friendship, the family, and all the pleasures of the experience to be more important than just eating. The food certainly counts, but let it be only one part of your total enjoyment. Even in a fast-food restaurant, you can choose to *dine*, or you can eat to get the food down and be done with it.

But I Paid for It!

Herein lies the biggest eating-out problem for some overweight people: they feel obliged to eat everything served. They think, "If I paid for it, you bet I'm going to eat it." They think that if they don't eat all of the food served, they're wasting money.

This thinking is terrifically fattening. The hunger scale of 0–5 goes out the window after the food arrives because, well, all good eating intentions disappear. Instead, the diner *consciously overeats* to avoid wasting money … then blames overeating on the amount of food served! This is like raising your hand and saying, "Over here! I'll pay you to help me get fatter!" It's just crazy.

If you've tended to think this way, please forgive yourself and resolve to change. If you don't, you won't be able to eat out and also reach your ideal size.

Here are some incredibly simple ways to improve your eating-out style:

1. **Eat enough (that is, eat up to 5 on the hunger scale) and take the rest home.** Leftovers can be a real treat and can stretch your food dollars. Never be embarrassed to ask for a take-home box. It's a thin thing to do.

2. **Share your meal with a friend.** Couples can regularly share meals, and perhaps you can share a meal with some of your friends, too. The waitperson seldom bats an eyelash, even in the fanciest restaurant. Order an extra salad or side vegetable if you want. Sharing an entrée also makes it easier to save room in your stomach for dessert.

3. **Think of eating out as entertainment.** View the food as just part of the total experience. That way, if you have a great time and only eat part of your meal, you'll still get your money's worth.

4. **Leave food on your plate.** Convince yourself that it's "cool" and enlightened not to eat everything you are served. It certainly is more of a thin way of eating.

> **CAUTION**
>
> **Weighty Warning**
>
> Don't let the quantity of food served or the attitude of a waitperson determine how you eat. The people who own, operate, or work at a restaurant aren't responsible for your weight. Only you are. Make sure that you're in charge when you eat out.

Be a Picky Eater

Be a picky eater in a restaurant, just as you would at home. By focusing on quality, not quantity, you're putting the emphasis on taste, not bulk. The shift in focus will help you slow down and enjoy your food more.

Order exactly what you want prepared exactly as you want it. If your favorite salad dressing is olive oil and vinegar with blue cheese crumbles, ask for just that. If you want your meat rare, ask for it rare. Don't be shy. You're paying.

If the food doesn't meet your standards, don't eat it. If you want to send it back to the kitchen, do so. Heck, if you want a certain pasta dish without the pasta, the cook can probably figure it out. Be polite but steadfast. After all, it's your tummy, your waistline, and your money we're talking about here.

Consume the Basics

In eating out, make sure that you follow the New Food Pyramid suggested in Chapter 12. It shouldn't be hard, even in ethnic restaurants. Every culture of the world eats proteins, carbohydrates, and fats. You should be able to find combinations of the three basic food groups that work for your body.

In choosing a restaurant, ask yourself these three questions:

1. Is my stomach now at 0? If not, can I be at 0 by the time we eat? When you don't start at 0, it will be harder to lose weight and may prevent you from staying at your ideal size.

2. Can I get at least 15 grams of high-quality complete protein in my meal at this restaurant? Fifteen grams is a portion about the size of a deck of cards. You

should be able to eat at virtually any restaurant in the world, with the possible exception of vegetarian restaurants, and get enough high-quality complete protein. At one of our favorite noodle restaurants, we order extra meat for our salad or pasta so we get enough.

3. Can I order enough vegetables and fruits? This is usually easy at regular sit-down restaurants and now at many fast-food restaurants. They offer salads, fruit, and salad bars.

Eating Breakfast Out

Breakfasts belong in a class by themselves. Your food selection is critical for daylong high energy. If you don't consume good fuel at breakfast, you can't expect to have a great day. Here's some advice for eating smart breakfasts out.

Fortunately, restaurant breakfast menus list foods with plenty of protein and usually some kind of fruit. Choose the high-quality protein foods (such as ham, Canadian bacon, and eggs) that will help you avoid the late-afternoon slumps that lead to overeating. Regular bacon is a marginally acceptable food because it is highly processed and filled with nitrates. That usually goes for pork products and turkey bacon, too.

Here are some of your better choices for restaurant breakfast food:

- Eggs with ham or steak
- Fresh fruit or fresh-squeezed juice
- Omelets
- Bacon (marginally acceptable)

- Eggs benedict
- Cheeses
- Vegetables
- Yogurt

Lean Lingo

The word **breakfast** is derived from the Middle English word *brek* (meaning "to break") plus fast from the old Norse word *fasta* (meaning "to fast"). Thus, when you eat your first meal of the day, you break your fast—no matter what time it is.

Poorer choices include the following:

- High-glycemic starches such as pancakes, muffins, bagels, scones, waffles, toast, English muffins, and donuts
- High-glycemic cereals, which is pretty much all of them with the exception of steel-cut oatmeal and barley
- Sausage

The poorer choices aren't "evil foods," but don't rely on them as breakfast staples. If you really want pancakes, however, order your eggs or meat and one or two small pancakes. Use real butter and savor thoroughly.

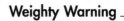

Weighty Warning

At a breakfast buffet, brunch, or other buffet-type meal, selectively choose what to put on your plate. Under no circumstances should you return to your table with a plate so loaded up that it looks like the foothills of the Rocky Mountains!

Breakfast buffets are challenging because of the variety and unusual food selections. You can become dazzled by the beautiful array of food and forget that your stomach is only as big as your fist. An all-you-can-eat buffet is the perfect opportunity to practice picky eating, enjoy the pleasures of eating beautifully, and not worry about maximizing how much food you're getting for your money. After all, why would you want to eat all that you can? It sounds fattening and uncomfortable.

So here's how to eat at a buffet. Even before you pick up your plate, walk around and check out the entire array of foods. Select which foods you definitely want to eat and which ones to pass on. If you see a dessert you really want, take it into account. As you go through the line with your plate, take only modest portions of the foods you really want.

Sit down, eat slowly, and enjoy your food. If the food doesn't taste as good as it looked, don't eat it. Eat up to 5. If you haven't reached 5, then and only then go back for seconds. You'll be thrilled with this approach.

Best Bets for Lunch and Dinner

Three types of restaurants are usually quite reliable for eating out appropriately—that is, for getting enough protein, fruits, and vegetables.

Steak Houses

Steak houses abound in most cities and towns. Typically, the selection is focused on— you guessed it—steak. Sometimes seafood, too. You can easily make smart meal choices. Many offer salad bars or fabulous salads. If you make sure to eat 0–5, you can have a great meal that keeps you moving toward reaching your ideal size.

Best menu choices include the following:

- Steak or prime rib with visible fat cut off
- Seafood or fish
- Vegetable of the day
- Sautéed mushrooms

- Salad bar or salad
- Baked sweet potato with butter (these are low-glycemic)
- Béarnaise sauce on veggies or meat
- Dessert of cheesecake or crème brûlée

Poorer choices include the following:

- White baked potato, especially if you plan to eat it all rather than a bite or two

- Anything starchy on the menu such as pasta
- Lots of bread

Since the size of the meals at steak houses can be large, they're a great place for sharing a meal. Or plan to bring leftovers home. That leftover steak makes a great and quick breakfast the next day.

Hamburgers, Ribs, and Such

These are usually low- to mid-priced, sit-down restaurants. Examples include Bennigan's, Tony Roma's, and Chili's. They offer you wonderful choices for eating to attain your ideal size.

Best menu choices include the following:

- Burgers (hold the bun) and maybe a few fries
- Meat entrées such as chicken, ribs, and steaks

- Dinner salads and side salads
- Fish and seafood
- Sandwiches—preferably hold the bread

Poorer choices include the following:

- Pasta dishes
- Sandwiches if you eat the bread

As you are beginning to notice, you can eat at any restaurant. Your food selections and eating 0–5 are what make you successful at getting to your ideal size.

Fresh Fish Houses

Any time you can eat fresh fish and seafood, go for it.

Good choices include the following:

- Fish and seafood entrées and appetizers

- Salads and veggies

- Butter, cocktail sauce, garlic sauce, or other condiments

- Sourdough bread (limit your consumption to a small piece)

Poorer choices include the following:

- Pasta dishes, which are seldom served al dente

- Too many French fries or too much baked potato

- Heavily breaded fish

> **Body of Knowledge**
>
> Because fish, especially salmon, contains essential fatty acids, you'll benefit from eating more. Fish and other seafood are excellent sources of high-quality protein.

Fast-Food Restaurants

Obviously, you don't go to a fast-food restaurant for gourmet dining (at least, we hope not!). But we assume you eat at them every now and then. We do, too. They're convenient, inexpensive, and fast. You don't have to give up going to fast-food restaurants to reach your ideal size, but you do need to eat smart. For starters, ignore the "fast-food" label. Eat just as slowly as you do at other meals so that you taste the food, digest it well, and feel your hunger numbers—before, during, and afterward.

The Usual Drive-Thru's or Eat-In's

Good choices at burger and chicken places include the following:

- Hamburger or cheeseburger (preferably toss the bun and eat the rest with a plastic fork)

- Salad

- Fried chicken (preferably remove the skin)

- Fried fish, hold the bun

- Orange juice

- Fresh fruit

- Coleslaw

Poorer choices include the following:

- French fries
- Milk shakes
- Diet sodas, colas, and pop
- Anything supersized

Delis and Sandwich Shops

These offer fast food with some interesting and healthy choices. Good choices include the following:

- Whole-wheat or low-carb wraps filled with meat, cheese, and lots of fresh veggies such as tomatoes, lettuce, cucumber, green peppers, and onions, as well as condiments such as black olives, pickles, and jalapeño chiles. You can open the wrap and eat the insides with a plastic fork. Yummy.

- A meatball sandwich with all the veggies and condiments. Eat with a fork, hold the bread.

- Any sandwich, hold the bread, with a couple of potato chips and a pickle.

- A piece of fresh fruit.

Poorer choices include the following:

- Eating all the bread on a sub (way too many carbs and way too high-glycemic!)

Popular Specialty Eateries

Now let's talk about salad-bar restaurants and pizza parlors. Both are tricky to eat at healthfully and attain your ideal size.

Salad-Bar Restaurants

At these restaurants, you can choose from a wide offering of fresh fruits and vegetables that your body wants and needs. Plus, you get to select just exactly what you want to eat and how much. So what's not to like? The answer: the lack of enough high-quality complete protein.

Often you'll find sliced hard-boiled eggs and cheese, but salad bars seldom offer meat or fish. You'll find it hard to consume at least 15 grams of protein. You may be able to find shreds of meat or seafood in a pasta salad. Skip the white-flour pasta and baked white potatoes.

Good choices include the following:

- Fresh fruits and vegetables
- Protein offerings such as hard-boiled eggs, cheese, and meat toppings
- Olive oil and vinegar dressing
- Moderate amounts of salad dressings, meaning 2 to 3 tablespoons

Poorer choices include the following:

- Mayonnaise-based salads with pasta or potatoes
- Baked potatoes
- Starchy dessert offerings
- Loading up on salad dressing
- Low-fat salad dressings

> **CAUTION** **Weighty Warning**
>
> Right now, picture your plate when you've been through the salad bar line. Does it look like a colorful mountain capped with enough salad dressing to ski down? Oops. Not good. Some salad dressing is good, but too much is ridiculous.

Pizza

Pizza can be a big challenge when losing weight. It's the second most popular eating-out food behind burgers and for good reason—it smells great, it's a super treat, and it's easily served at everything from office luncheons to family parties. You even get to eat it with your fingers! Plus, it's only a quick phone call away. (P.S. Make sure that the local delivery number isn't on your speed dialer!)

You'll never get away from pizza, and we don't want you to think of it as an evil food, but how you eat pizza can make a big difference in releasing fat from your body. Here are four pizza-eating tips:

First, when you get to choose the toppings, pick the meats or fish—ham, hamburger, anchovies, and Canadian bacon—and add veggies or fruits. Avoid ordering double cheese.

Second, when you eat pizza, eat with a fork. Eat the topping and leave behind the crust, no matter whether the crust is deep dish or thin and crisp. Leave it for the trashcan. This could be a challenge but give it a try.

Third, when you can, order a side salad with the pizza. You'll then have a balanced meal.

Fourth, eat slowly and make sure that you eat 0–5. Don't even think about a third piece of pizza until you've stopped and checked with your body to see what your hunger number is.

Good choices include the following:

♦ Meat toppings (unfortunately pepperoni and sausage are the least desirable)

♦ Other vegetable and fruit toppings

♦ A side salad

Poorer choices include the following:

♦ Double cheese

♦ Highly-processed meat toppings such as pepperoni and sausage

♦ The crust

If anyone has the insensitivity to ask you why you aren't eating the crust, just shrug your shoulders lightly and say, "The toppings are so good, I just don't want the crust." This should end the conversation, unless the person asks for your leftover crust.

Ethnic Food

Yes, you can eat comfortably at ethnic restaurants and enjoy the interesting, varied, and delightful cuisines. Remember to (1) consume the types of foods that best nourish your body, and (2) eat 0–5.

Mexican Food

Olé! Mexican and Tex-Mex cuisines are delicious, and if you enjoy spicy foods and hot chilies, these restaurants are hard to resist. Often high-quality complete protein comes wrapped in a starch—either corn or wheat tortillas or corn meal, as with tamales. Consequently, it's best to eat less of the wrapping and more of the filling. This is the same as our sandwich recommendations.

Thinspiration

If you really love the taste of the salsa that comes with the corn chips served before your meal at Mexican restaurants, it is fine to eat the salsa with a spoon and bypass all the chips. Salsa has great veggie value and great taste. It makes a great salad dressing, too!

Good choices include the following:

♦ Guacamole dip (avocados are especially healthy and good for weight loss)

♦ Salsa with some corn chips

♦ Tortilla soup

- Carne adobada, or marinated long-cooked pork

- Carnitas

- Tamales, tacos, enchiladas, burritos, chimichangas, and other "wrapped" meat mixtures

- Salads

- Taco salad

- Fajitas

- Beans

- For dessert, flan (if you have room)

Poorer choices include the following:

- Overeating the chips before the entrée arrives

- Eating all the rice or even most of it

- Ordering cheese rather than meat or chicken fillings

- Sopapillas for dessert (they're just fried bread)

You may find Mexican food so delightful that it's hard to stop eating at 5. Be sure to eat slowly so that you enjoy all the flavors; otherwise, it can seem as if 5 comes too soon.

Italian Restaurants

Even Italian food can help you get to your ideal size. Italian food isn't just pasta and breads; it includes fabulous meat and seafood dishes. Think veal piccata or scaloppini. Think fried calamari or mussels in a wine garlic sauce. Think fresh, sliced tomatoes with mozzarella and basil. Yes, you certainly can get a balanced meal and eat healthy at your favorite Italian eatery.

Good choices include the following:

- Beef, poultry, veal, fish, pork, and seafood entrées and appetizers

- Fresh salads such as Caesar and garden salads

- Small side dishes of pasta

- Fresh fruit, canolis, or cheesecake for dessert

- Extra meatballs with spaghetti

Poorer choices include the following:

◆ Pasta

◆ Fettuccine alfredo

◆ Filling up on bread and pasta

Bring home what you can't eat. Meatballs make a great breakfast, as do other entrée choices.

Asian Restaurants

Asian cuisine is quite varied and, in this section, includes Chinese, Vietnamese, Korean, Thai, and others. The same fundamentals apply here as to eating out in general. Make sure that you get enough protein and fresh fruits and vegetables.

CAUTION

Weighty Warning

Watch out for the huge portions served at Asian restaurants. Instead, stop when your stomach is comfortable before you are full and take the leftovers home, asking the waitperson to wrap the rice separately from the rest of the food. Or better yet, don't take the leftover rice home.

Sometimes when you eat a dish that's stir-fried, it can be hard to judge whether you've had enough protein. It's one reason why so many people feel hungry soon after eating oriental food. They seemed to eat plenty, but the food didn't contain enough high-quality protein to keep their engine stoked and their metabolism high.

Many Asian restaurants use MSG—monosodium glutamate—as a flavor enhancer for their food. We recommend that you always ask the waitperson to keep it out of your food.

Good choices include the following:

◆ Meat-, fish-, and seafood-based dishes. (Make sure that they contain more than just shreds of meat; they should have enough to make up an amount the size of a deck of cards.)

◆ Stir-fried vegetables or vegetable side dishes. (Some oriental vegetable dishes are terrific.)

◆ A taste of rice or noodles, but not a plateful.

◆ The soups, provided they don't contain MSG.

Poorer choices include the following:

♦ Filling up on rice or noodles

♦ Stir-fried rice—too much starch, too little protein

♦ Anything with MSG in it

♦ Your fortune cookie (Read the fortune and pass on the starchy cookie.)

French Restaurants

French cuisine in general offers excellently balanced meals and delicious food. Most often, the meals are made with fresh ingredients and don't contain preservatives and artificial ingredients.

Good choices include the following:

♦ Meat, seafood, fish, and poultry entrées

♦ Vegetables and salads

♦ Desserts—crème brûlée, mousse, and cheesecake

Poorer choices include the following:

♦ Eating too much of that great French bread

♦ Eating quickly without savoring

♦ Too much French wine

Other Ethnic Cuisines

No matter what the cuisine, whether it's Middle Eastern, German, Russian, South American, Indian, or any other, you can eat in ways that encourage your body to release weight if you follow these guidelines:

♦ Eat only when you are hungry, at 0.

♦ Stop eating at or below being satisfied, meaning at or below 5.

Thinspiration

No food is so powerful that it can make you fat. But by eating with wisdom, every food you eat—no matter what type—can support your weight loss and weight maintenance.

◆ Make sure that you eat enough high-quality complete protein, at least 15 grams.

◆ Make sure that you get at least one serving of fruit or vegetables and preferably two.

◆ Avoid eating high-glycemic starches.

The Least You Need to Know

◆ Eating out is part of life, and you can eat out by ordering regular foods with the confidence that you are getting to your ideal size.

◆ Ordering from the menu is easy when you order what you want and also what offers a healthy balance of protein, carbohydrates, and fats.

◆ You can dine beautifully without drawing attention to your eating and still reach your ideal size.

◆ Sharing meals when you eat out and bringing home leftovers make sense for your budget and your size.

◆ All cuisines are friendly and can support you in getting to your ideal size when you know how to order and eat.

Chapter 28

Special Occasion Eating

In This Chapter

- Eating for the holidays
- Family eating situations
- Celebrating with ease and confidence
- Handling weight-loss comments

Holidays and special occasions can now be enjoyable rather than fattening. No longer do you need to fear the holiday season and packing on 5 to 10 extra pounds. This also means you won't be writing New Year's resolutions to lose weight! You can sail through the holidays—as well as vacations and special occasions such as weddings—with confidence, knowing that you are moving steadily toward your ideal size.

The Tradition of Feasting

Feasting on special occasions has been around about as long as mankind. Why? Because we like to honor life's rites of passage and religious celebrations, and what better way than to have a party that includes special foods. Feasting days through the ages have included religious holidays, life event celebrations such as marriages and births, season changes, and sporting events, just like today.

Thinspiration

If you have favorite feast foods, such as cranberry sauce or rum balls, remember that you can enjoy them at other times of the year as well. This might relieve some of the subtle internal pressure to fill up at the celebration because you won't see that special food again for another year.

In days of old, common folk ate pretty boring and simple foods from day to day. Their meager diet included some meat, in-season vegetables and fruits, and starches such as bread or rice. Their diet might also include a soupy cereal called gruel ... which even sounds boring.

But feast days were different. The English and American colonists would celebrate by making and eating all sorts of delicacies like plum pudding, mince meat pies, and yes, even fruitcake. (Imagine a bleak, cold winter without any fresh produce. Now take some fruit that was dried or preserved since the summer, add nuts, and bake them into a cake. Fruitcake would have seemed like a delicacy to you, too.) These feast days might have been the only times when the common folk had access to fancy "treat" foods.

The common folk could afford to overindulge at a feast because they seldom, if ever, had enough food, let alone enough to constantly overeat.

Now jump to the present. You don't face food scarcity from day to day. Eating enough calories to fuel your body is as easy as reaching into the pantry or the refrigerator or stopping by a fast-food joint. Finding special foods is easy, too. What you can't find at a local store, you can order over the Internet and have delivered directly to your home.

Yet, you still want to enjoy special feasts. The good news is that if you update your perspective about feasts, you can enjoy special foods without overeating them. But to get through feasts with your waistline slim, it takes some thought and planning.

Thinspiration

Cooking a whole turkey isn't a requirement for Thanksgiving; it's just a tradition. You could also cook other foods such as a roast or a ham. Don't feel compelled to make all the trimmings. Be selective and prepare only the foods you and your family enjoy the most.

Thanksgiving

Thanksgiving has to be the biggest overeating day in the United States. Our custom is to prepare a turkey with all the trimmings, and the trimmings often include lots of high-glycemic foods such as mashed potatoes, stuffing, and bread. Plus, our informal custom is to have candy, cheese and crackers, and cookies available all day long. Even just a taste of each of the trimmings can leave a person well above 5 on the hunger scale.

After we learned to hate the feeling of being really full, we devised a Thanksgiving eating strategy. It's pretty simple:

1. Make sure that you are at 0 on the hunger scale before you sit down to dinner. This might mean passing up the appetizers and treats scattered around the house. Save those treats for later or the next day.

2. Only put on your plate modest portions of the foods you like the very best. (Perhaps you prefer dark meat, cranberry sauce, and dressing. Yes, this is an unbalanced meal, but just on this day you can afford it.)

3. Save room for dessert if you like the dessert. In other words, pumpkin pie is great only if you like it.

4. Don't worry about hurting anyone's feelings if you don't eat food they prepared. If the person insists you take some, put the food on your plate, eat one bite, and as you eat, hide the rest under something else!

5. Say a blessing. After all, this is Thanksgiving.

6. Eat slowly and try to make this meal last at least 30 minutes. Many families, when they finally sit down to eat their feast, gulp it down, sometimes in order to not miss the next football game. Bad idea.

7. Eat 0–5.

8. Don't go back for seconds unless your hunger number is below 5. The leftovers can be eaten the next day and even the day after that … and the day after that … and so on.

9. Have a conversation plan. Perhaps everyone at the table can say what he or she gives thanks for. Make it a fun, upbeat, and bonding time.

Be sure to focus your energy on the purpose of the celebration and the togetherness of family and friends. Let the food be a part of the celebration, not the purpose of the celebration.

Happy Holidays ... Really

You can breeze through the holiday season, that time between Thanksgiving and New Year's Day, and even lose weight or stay at your ideal size. And while you breeze through, you can still enjoy the special foods and treats of the season.

Sound too good to be true? It *is* possible. Other people do it. Basically, successful holiday eaters, whether they consciously know it or not, eat from 0–5. So can you, but it takes some planning. You are presented with so many opportunities to eat fabulous foods—family parties, office parties, office treats, cocktail parties, open houses, cookie exchanges, and so on. You could go through the holidays without ever feeling a simple hunger pang.

Don't be discouraged. Here are some helpful hints to get you through the season smiling:

- Always start eating at 0.

- Go easy on the alcohol. Drinking alcohol can impair your ability to feel your stomach's hunger number. Alcoholic beverages increase your body's production of the stress hormone, cortisol, which causes abdominal weight gain.

- Take small tastes of food rather than real portions at parties.

- Make sure that you get at least 15 grams of protein at meals. The protein can come in the form of hors d'oeuvres, such as shrimp on toothpicks or bacon-wrapped liver.

- Don't taste or eat everything offered. Party foods are not precious rarities. You'll have other opportunities to eat them.

- Focus on enjoying the people, the conversation, and the ambience. After all, you're at a party.

- Make the party and the people more important than the food.

- If you have multiple parties on the same day, you might want to eat only to a hunger number of 2 or 3 at each party so that you can sample food at each event.

- Always, always stop eating at or below 5 on the hunger scale.

- Maintain your exercise program throughout the holidays.

- Spend time remembering the true meaning of the holidays.

Thinspiration

Since the holidays occur during the dark time of the year in the northern hemisphere, when the sun rises late and sets early, some people get the blues from sunlight deprivation. Make sure that you get out in the sunshine if you can or use a light box as a source of mood-lifting, full-spectrum light.

Home Alone for the Holidays

Being alone or almost alone for the holidays can be fattening. It's easy to feel left out and sorry for yourself. Don't console yourself with food. You can still share the joys of the holidays with others and yourself. Here are a few suggestions:

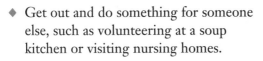

Thinspiration

The difference between being alone and being lonely is your state of mind. Do whatever it takes to enjoy yourself and to avoid having a personal pity party.

◆ Get out and do something for someone else, such as volunteering at a soup kitchen or visiting nursing homes.

◆ Go to church, mosque, synagogue, or temple and be with other people.

◆ Take quality time for yourself. Pamper, polish, exercise, read, and catch up with your projects and yourself.

◆ Eat with wisdom, like you've now learned to do every day. Eat 0–5.

◆ Savor some special holiday treats, but carefully and sensuously.

Parties

Whether you're at a dinner party, a wedding, a Super Bowl celebration, or a neighborhood potluck, apply the same eating principles:

Weighty Warning

Because of the nature of potlucks, sometimes you might find very little high-quality protein offered. To make sure that you get enough protein, maybe you should be the one to bring a protein dish. Foods such as sliced roast or ham, deviled eggs, and a lovely presentation of cheese and fruit make a terrific contribution.

◆ Make the party, the celebration, and the people more important than the food.

◆ Start eating at 0 on the hunger scale.

◆ Be selective about what foods you put on your plate.

◆ Eat slowly, carefully, and sensuously.

◆ Save room for dessert or wedding cake if you want some.

◆ Drink alcohol with caution, remembering that it dulls your hunger sensations, making it tough to know when you've had enough food.

◆ Stop eating at or below 5.

Learn how to be socially comfortable at parties so that you can have a good time without hiding out near the appetizer tray. If you need to, take a class on small talk or lessons in the art of party going. Such classes really exist, and they can be quite helpful.

Handling Family and Friends

Why does it seem that people push food on you more when you're on a program to master your weight? Some family events can be emotionally challenging all by themselves; you sure don't need anyone telling you how to eat.

In many families, food is a representation of love. Therefore, a host or hostess might assume his or her love is not accepted if you don't eat enough food in that person's opinion. Herein lies a big problem. You know that food is not love—at least you should by now—but try explaining that at a family event. It's bound to upset the fun.

Thinspiration

When someone suggests that you're becoming too thin, thank the person for his or her concern and keep your own counsel. Since you are being successful at losing weight, you can consider it to be a compliment. Your risk of becoming anorexic is miniscule to nonexistent. Only if your body mass index drops below 18 do you need to be concerned.

The best way to navigate through this minefield at a family gathering is to keep your own counsel. Keep quiet about your weight-loss program. If anyone mentions it, thank the person for noticing and change the subject. If you're done eating and someone is pushing you to eat more, simply tell the person that you don't have any more room or that you might have some more food later after your food settles. Then you can politely refuse more food later if it's offered.

The Least You Need to Know

♦ We live in an age of abundance in which special foods formerly reserved for feasts are widely available every day at food stores and over the Internet.

♦ At special events, focus on the celebration and not the food.

♦ Overeating during the holidays and at parties is not a requirement; in fact, you can continue to lose weight and enjoy the parties.

♦ Be prepared to handle comments from family and friends about your new weight and new ways of eating.

Chapter 29

The Support You Need

In This Chapter

- ◆ Finding the right support group
- ◆ Creating your own group
- ◆ Celebrating wins
- ◆ Supporting yourself

People who lose weight in groups tend to lose more weight and maintain their new sizes more easily. The mutual support and encouragement helps you tackle the challenges and keeps you going through the ups and downs of reaching your ideal size.

Needing support is normal. By nature, on our journeys through life, we seek companionship and soul mates. Your journey to reach your ideal size is no different. A personal support group can be a huge help. Its members are your cheerleaders, a sounding board, and a place to discuss your eating concerns. Whether your support group is just one other person or 20, being part of a group can make a difference in your success. The good news is that going the distance alone isn't necessary.

Support Helps

As you know already from experience, losing weight presents many potential roadblocks and some difficult terrain. We're referring to such things as late-night eating binges or unconsciously polishing off the whole bucket of popcorn at the movie. Perhaps in a nervous social setting, you might chomp down on dozens of appetizers or experience emotional upheaval that leads you to drown your sorrows in a quart of ice cream!

> **Thinspiration**
>
> If a weight-loss support group fits you, join and stay with it. If it doesn't fit, find another option. A support group that doesn't fit is like a shoe that's too small. No matter what you do, it still isn't going to fit. You don't need to bend and conform so that you can fit into the weight-loss group.

Then there's the question of how to emotionally deal with the slip-ups, the little binges, the eating past 5 on the hunger scale. Picking yourself back up and rebuilding your weight-loss resolve can be challenging. Some days it can seem easier to just give up and forget about trying to get to your ideal size.

You don't have to do it alone. Let's repeat that: you don't have to do it alone. A support group can give you the encouragement to keep on keeping on—one day at a time or one phone call at a time until you reach your ideal size.

Support groups come in many varieties. Here are some of your choices:

- **Formal commercially sponsored groups.** These are usually part of national weight-loss programs such as Weight Watchers. Meetings cost about $10 per session and are based on the eating philosophy of the sponsor. But beware. You might have to step on the scale or do other unproductive activities, so preview the group before you join. If you don't feel positively motivated after your first couple meetings, don't go back.

- **Internet support from such sites as eDiets and iVillage.** Since the Internet is perpetually available, you can sign on at any time for information and encouragement. Many of these sites have ongoing chat rooms. Some offer online consultations with registered dietitians and psychologists. (Lucy's website at www.LucyBeale. com and Sandy's website at www. NutritionSandy.com offer information and e-mail support.)

- **Ongoing groups in your town.** These groups are often listed on community bulletin boards and in the local newspapers. Sometimes attendance is free, sometimes not.

◆ **A group sponsored by a weight-loss coach, registered dietitian, or by your church.** Most likely there's a fee for these groups, but it can be money well spent.

◆ **Your own support group.** You can form your own small group of friends or acquaintances that meets together for lunch, dinner, at each other's homes, or virtually via the Internet. You'll learn more about this in the next section.

Make sure that the support group you choose is uplifting and positive. In some groups, people become very emotional and delve into their heavy-duty life conditions and challenges. Decide whether that feels good to you and, most of all, whether it ultimately supports you in getting to your ideal size. Don't get hooked into a group that's little more than a gripe-whine session.

In addition, when choosing a support group, be sure to attend about three sessions to find out how it feels and whether it meets your needs. Use the following criteria for your decision:

◆ Are the people in the group dealing with many of the same eating and weight issues that you are?

◆ Do the people in the group have about the same amount of weight to lose as you do?

◆ Are the group members losing weight or just talking about it?

◆ Is the flow of the conversation uplifting and positive?

◆ Do the group members really want to get to their ideal size, and are they willing to do what it takes?

◆ Are you comfortable with the weight-loss and eating philosophies presented?

◆ Are the members celebrating their wins at each meeting and getting positive acknowledgement and reinforcement for their progress?

If the group feels right, join it and be an active participant so that you take away something from the meetings and make progress toward your goals. If the time comes when you need to move on, do so. It's perfectly fine to leave the group when it no longer meets your needs. Don't ever let yourself be shamed into staying by the group leader or by the other members.

Create Your Support Group

Putting together and orchestrating a support group is an excellent way for you to reach your goals, especially if you're willing to remain the group leader. When you devote the time and energy to help the group succeed, you'll accelerate reaching your ideal size and staying there.

First, determine what you want for your group in terms of time, cost, number of people, forms of interaction, and eating and weight philosophy. Since you already know plenty of people who also want to get to their ideal size, let them know you want to start a group. Set up the format and guidelines and get started.

Here are some suggestions for the format:

◆ **Weekly meetings in person.** To succeed, group members must really commit to get to the meetings. The advantage is that you support each other's weight-loss efforts from week to week, and you'll literally see how others are doing. That, in itself, can be motivating. If weekly face-to-face meetings are inconvenient or take too much time, use the phone.

◆ **Weekly meetings on the phone.** Conference call or set up a daisy chain using three-way calling. These meetings are easy to get to—they're as close as your phone—and can be done from virtually anywhere. It's a good idea for your group to get together in person every month or at least every other month.

◆ **Live online chat.** Your group can schedule to "meet" via the Internet at the same time. Generally speaking, if you're willing to schedule an e-mail chat, you might as well schedule a phone meeting, but an Internet group meeting might meet some groups' needs. An added benefit is that you won't have any long-distance bills.

◆ **Frequent e-mail contact.** This is excellent for between-meeting contact and follow-up. If you add a threaded-discussion format, you can follow and discuss topics over time.

◆ **One-on-one phone calls for emergencies.** The group members can exchange telephone numbers and agree to call each other for support. A support call helps soothe the feelings of isolation and fear that occur when a person is highly stressed, overeats, and even when he or she wants to binge.

In support groups, people come and go, so be prepared to accept the flow and continue to invite others to join your group. People who are losing weight tend to be skittish about such things as accountability, progress, and bumps along the way. Some will drop out. Keep the group upbeat about losing and adding members.

The Group Agenda

Support groups are effective when the members are getting results and when they are finding solutions to their eating problems. Plus, seeing group members lose weight motivates others to do the same, as in "If she can do it, so can I."

Keep the meetings flowing and fun. In about one hour, people can get support, develop camaraderie, and leave feeling motivated.

Here's a suggested agenda:

- **Open with an inspirational quote or saying.**

- **Celebrate wins.** Have each person share his or her wins for the week. If this takes too long, have each person write down their 10 wins for the week, pair up, and share in pairs. Acknowledge each other for the wins. It doesn't matter how big or small the win; what matters is that wins are acknowledged. Ooh and aah about everyone's wins and successes. Applaud. We all need this.

- **Address problems and solutions.** Give each person the opportunity to present any roadblocks encountered during the past week. The group can brainstorm solutions. This way, everyone in the group learns to think creatively about eating and emotional situations, and they learn how to change their behavior and attitudes.

- **Introduce educational items.** Each week a different person can present new information about nutrition, exercise, or research on weight loss. Occasionally invite a guest speaker, such as an exercise expert or nutritionist.

- **Commit for the upcoming week.** Each person makes a personal commitment to his or her action plan for the next week. The weekly action plan includes exercise, eating, affirmations, and general goal setting.

- **Offer a thought for the week.** Make it an inspirational or fun moment.

> **Body of Knowledge**
>
> As with other important parts of your life, writing down your weekly weight-loss action plan will help you get it done. There's something about committing plans to paper that gives the tasks more focus and boosts your determination. Your written plan can include your goals, the key steps you're planning to follow, and some way to mark off or record your wins.

Consider sharing the responsibility for managing the group and meetings with several other people. That way, those who share group leadership become more committed to everyone's success, which, in turn, will motivate them toward personal success as well.

Going It Alone

If groups don't fit for you, create your own personal support system. You can even hold your own meeting with yourself. At a minimum, once a week take the time to assess your progress. You can even follow the preceding agenda.

Make sure that you celebrate your wins. A win can be a big thing, such as fitting into a smaller pair of jeans, or it can be something small. An example of a win is not overeating when you go out to dinner or passing up the donuts at the office because you weren't at 0 on the hunger scale. Write your wins down either daily or weekly so that you have written proof of your progress. All wins are significant. They represent the steps you've taken toward reaching your ideal size.

Thinspiration

Celebrating weight-loss wins sets you up for more and more success. Review your day and your week in terms of what you accomplished, not based on what you left undone or the mistakes made. View your journey to your ideal size from the perspective of the hero's path. The mere undertaking of mastering your weight and your eating makes you a hero or heroine.

At your personal progress meeting with yourself, work out your weekly action plan. Schedule your exercise sessions for the next week. You might even make a grocery list to stock up on the foods you most enjoy that fit your nutrition plan. Look ahead to any parties and celebrations and plan your approach. For example, plan how to arrive already at 0, what to wear, and how to have the most enjoyable time.

Finally, keep your motivation strong by using positive self-talk and by finding quotes or information on how to keep your resolve and commitment strong. You might even reread chapters in this book that will reinvigorate your determination.

The Least You Need to Know

- People in weight-loss support groups tend to lose more weight and more easily stay at their ideal size.

- Whether you join a commercial support group, a group in your community, or an online version, check it out first to make sure that it works for you and meets your needs.

- You can hold your own support meeting with yourself to support your progress and stay on track toward attaining your ideal size.

Chapter 30

Maintaining Your Ideal Size

In This Chapter

- ◆ Solidifying your success
- ◆ Writing your good-bye, fat-self letter
- ◆ Moving beyond your weight issue
- ◆ Responding if you gain a few pounds
- ◆ Dressing at your ideal size

Maintaining your weight loss involves many, many aspects of your life. Certainly what and how you eat make a big difference in staying at your ideal size, but how you think and how you live are also important.

You want to be truly finished with being overweight. Permanently. Forever. You don't want any part of your former overweight self hanging around as you live the rest of your life. You want the "new you" to be "the real you" for the rest of your life.

Sometimes formerly overweight individuals constantly fret about food and dieting. They can't seem to let go of the issue. We don't want that to happen with you. When your weight loss is complete, when you reach your ideal size, it's time (with a capital T) for you to bid a fond farewell to your fat self and get on with other, more interesting aspects of life.

The Good-Bye, Fat Self Letter

Write a good-bye letter to your fat self. To sign and seal the deal, write a good old-fashioned "Dear John" letter. Declare to your fat self that the relationship is over—*finis!*—and that you're starting a new life with your thin self.

Are you ready? Then let's do it. Set aside 15 minutes to a half-hour and, using pen and paper, write your letter. Tell your fat self that you appreciate all it has done for you. Thank it for all of the lessons it presented to you. Acknowledge all the lessons learned along the way.

Thinspiration

Try writing a good-bye, fat self letter even before you have reached your ideal size. You might be surprised at how hard it is to really say good-bye, but doing so early on can help you align your mindset with your goals.

Tell your fat self that you won't be needing it any longer for protection and padding, that you have found other ways to meet those needs. Then say a fond good-bye and let your fat self go.

Read the letter aloud and, if you want, create a ceremony (such as lighting a candle) to say your formal good-byes. Then release your fat self forever and welcome in your new ideal size.

Your good-bye letter to your fat self should be as personal as possible, but we're including a brief sample to help you get started:

Dear Fat Self,

You're going to find this hard to believe, but it's finally time for us to part ways. Forever. We've been together for __ years, through good times and bad, through thick and, well, not exactly thin. But the relationship is over. I don't plan to be over-weight ever again. You taught me a lot about life and about myself. Now I know how to eat and live without you.

You brought me lots of pain, too. Because of you, I've been unhappy. I've been through more clothes sizes than I care to think about. You've made shopping unpleas-ant. You've made food seem like some evil that I couldn't resist. You've made me cry. You've even made my health worse. I'm tired of it. It's over. I will not—repeat, NOT—be a fat person ever again. I'm much happier at my ideal size. I look better, feel better, and know I'm healthier. I plan to ignore that I ever knew you. So, adios. Sayonara. Auf wiedersehen. Good-bye!

Your good-bye letter can cover very specific issues to which you want to say good-bye. You can itemize the pains you've personally experienced and the past frustrations you've had trying to lose weight. To further solidify letting go of your previous fat self, we recommend that you use the exercise in the next section.

Thinspiration

What do you do if you're stuck at a certain size and your weight just won't budge? Write a good-bye letter to that size. In the letter, ask to be given all the lessons from your current size so that you can move on to the next size. We've seen people lose a size within days of writing this letter.

Moving Beyond

Letting go of your fatter self should be easy, shouldn't it? Not necessarily. Even though you didn't like being overweight, it was familiar to you. The truth is, you and your overweight self spent lots of time together. You were, after all, on an intimate first-name basis.

This exercise lets you finally cut the ties that bind you to that old persona. Using the exercise, you'll complete a quick makeover that will put you emotionally, mentally, and spiritually in sync with your ideal size.

The "Moving Beyond" Exercise Steps

Here's how it works. Give yourself a half-hour or more and, with notepad and pen in hand, do the following:

◆ On the top of the first page write, "Why I am thankful for having had a weight issue." List what you learned and whatever else comes to mind. List items such as protection, padding, and avoidance of hard choices.

◆ On the next page write, "What I leave behind with my weight issue." Save space to list any personality qualities you want to leave behind, along with activities, big-size clothing, relationships, and so on. Be sure to add overeating to the list, as well as telling yourself that you're fat.

◆ On the third page write, "Who I forgive and why." Be sure to include yourself. List people you know as well as media figures and magazines that have made you feel bad or have affected your eating behavior. You can even forgive fast-food restaurants for introducing the "supersize" meal!

◆ On the fourth page write, "What I learned from having a weight issue." Some of your answers could be duplicates from the preceding lists, but keep on writing everything that comes to mind. For instance, you've now learned how to eat as a thin person, how to master your weight, and how to take good care of yourself.

◆ On the fifth page write, "What I look forward to as I live at my ideal size." List your dreams, clothing, health, fitness level, activities, relationships, and career.

Take your time and fill out each page, listing your answers to the questions. Just write what comes to mind. It might take a while, so don't feel rushed. Then set an appointment with yourself for your "moving beyond" ceremony.

> **Body of Knowledge**
>
> In addition to helping you move beyond your weight issue, the "moving beyond" exercise will also work for other aspects of your life. You can use similar questions for changing jobs, changing relationships, selling your home, and even for finalizing the grieving process. We've seen people work small miracles of healing in their lives by using this simple and elegant exercise.

The "Moving Beyond" Ceremony

At your "moving beyond" ceremony, you can light candles, burn incense, go to a beautiful location, or do whatever pleases you. Then read your lists aloud and enjoy the feeling of release from your weight issue once and for all. Yes, you can even burn the pages at the end if that will add to your sense of completion.

The ceremony isn't just for show. Our clients who take the time to do the "moving beyond" exercise and ceremony are much more successful at staying at their ideal size. It empowers them to walk away with finality from any attachment they have to their former weightier selves. It solidifies their weight loss and their commitment to a new lighter self.

Part of your ceremony could include giving away overweight clothes to the thrift shop and paring down your wardrobe to fit your ideal size. Resolve never to need fat clothes again.

If Those Jeans Get Tight

If you ever find your jeans getting tight, you must take immediate action. We can't emphasize this enough. Don't procrastinate. Don't get depressed or anxious. Take action. It is a whole lot easier to lose 3 or 4 pounds than to lose 20. By taking immediate action, you should be able to fit into those jeans within 5 to 10 days, maybe by the next weekend!

Thinspiration

Most people's weight fluctuates from time to time. The secret to staying at your ideal size is to go directly back to the basics the minute your clothes feel too tight. Start eating 0–5, recording your intake, and doing your exercise program. Don't get seduced into quick-loss diet fads and gimmicks.

Gaining a couple of pounds happens to most people from time to time whether or not they were ever overweight. Short-term gain comes from overeating and also with age and stress.

Here's what to do when your clothes feel tight:

1. Start keeping a food diary that lists your beginning and ending hunger numbers. Record everything you put in your mouth except water.

2. Only eat when your stomach hunger number is 0 and stop eating when you're satisfied and before you're full—that is, stop at or below 5.

3. Make sure that you're getting a good balance of high-quality protein, fruits, and vegetables. (We also recommend consuming about two tablespoons of essential fatty acids daily.)

4. Keep up your exercise program. If you have stopped exercising, start again immediately and work up wisely to your former intensity levels of cardio, strength training, and stretching.

5. Consciously eat 0–5.

6. Start writing your affirmations again every day. Write, "I, (*fill in your name*), am now a naturally healthy and thin person. I wear a size (*insert ideal size*), and I do what thin people do." Write this in your notebook 10 times daily.

7. Use the stress reducers listed in Chapter 8 as a way to reduce stress and stop emotional eating.

8. Review other information in this book and make note of where you may have gotten off track. Then take positive action to correct your situation.

If you do the preceding, you can expect quick results. Your body at its ideal size has established a new set point, and it wants to stay there. So help it out. It will respond.

Dressing at Your Ideal Size

You're at your ideal size. At last you can wear all those fashionable clothes you've longed to wear. Perhaps you've noticed that people who are at their ideal size often wear different styles of clothing than people who are overweight. You have many more choices now that you've reached your ideal size. You'll never need to wear vertical stripes just because they make you look thinner—you are thinner!

We suggest that you reinforce your commitment to yourself by avoiding "overweight" types of clothes. Take a look at the following lists, and you'll get a sense of the clothing that will show off your new body.

In general, give up wearing these "overweight" clothing styles:

◆ Big and long shirts, over-blouses and tunics on men and women

◆ Elastic-stretch waistbands

◆ Stretch pants designed to accommodate weight gain

◆ Big, flowing dresses and slacks

◆ Tent-shaped dresses

◆ Big, loose, long, and flowing jackets or coats

◆ Clothing purchased in "big people" shops

◆ Huge sweatshirts

> **Body of Knowledge**
>
> If dressing as a thin person is new to you, enlist the help of a professional wardrobe coach or a knowledgeable salesperson. This type of person can help you coordinate your wardrobe so that your clothes meet your new lifestyle needs and you don't overspend your budget.

Instead, you might choose:

◆ Slacks with leather belts

◆ Tailored slacks and pantsuits

◆ Form-fitting stretch jeans

◆ T-shirts and torso-hugging knits

◆ Tailored blazers and jackets

◆ Shirts tucked into slacks or skirts or well-fitted tops over slacks (pass on the tunics and large overblouses)

- Shorter skirts when they're in style (and even when they aren't!)

- Sexy heels and sandals

- Sundresses and evening wear that show some skin

Choose clothing that tastefully and lovingly reveals rather than hides your body. You have done a lot of work to master your weight. It's perfectly fine to show off your success.

The Need for Compassion

You know firsthand the pain and sadness of being overweight. You also know the prejudice and ridicule you endured when you were bigger. So make a firm commitment to never look down on or criticize others who have yet to reach their ideal size. You owe it to yourself and, in a sense, to the world.

Thinspiration

Give the gifts of understanding and compassion to others who are still struggling with their weight issues. Follow the golden rule. Treat others just as you wish you had been treated when you were overweight.

No one should have to feel the pain of low self-esteem and prejudicial treatment because of his or her weight. Now that you've mastered your weight, you can be part of the solution, not part of the problem. Here are some suggestions for how to help others:

- Respect the challenges that others still face.

- Never become preachy about losing weight.

- Graciously accept compliments without gloating.

- Offer advice only when asked for it.

- When asked, let people know that they can master their weight.

Because you've mastered getting to your ideal size, you've demonstrated that the epidemic of obesity and being overweight can be solved—one person at a time. You've actually helped make the world a healthier place. If others ask how you mastered your weight issue, by all means share your success story so that you can help them experience the joy and freedom you now have. But be sure to do so graciously and kindly.

The Least You Need to Know

- Writing a good-bye letter to your fat self lets you solidify your weight-loss success.

- Use the "moving beyond" exercise to once and for all walk away from your weight issue.

- Should your jeans get tight, immediately get back on track by recording your food intake, eating 0–5, and using affirmations.

- Dress as a thin person to enhance your body; do not hide it.

- Direct the compassion and forgiveness you have developed toward yourself and your weight issue to others who are still struggling with their weight.

Glossary

adrenal glands   Two glands located in the stomach that produce hormones related to stress, including adrenaline and cortisol.

adrenaline   A hormone produced in response to stress that directly affects the brain as a stimulus. It is known as the fight-or-flight hormone.

affirmation   A positive statement declaring that you already have what you want.

amino acid   The basic unit that makes up protein. We must get essential amino acids from our food to maintain health. Nonessential amino acids can be synthesized in the body but are also required for health.

appetite   A natural biological desire for food that may vary daily.

autonomic nervous system   The part of the nervous system that controls involuntary responses in the body.

basal metabolism rate (BMR)   The number of calories your body needs for basic involuntary processes such as breathing, eyes blinking, heart beating, digesting, and so on.

bitter orange   An herb used in some diet supplements that has mild amphetaminelike stimulants.

body mass index (BMI)   A measure of the relationship between height and weight.

calorie   A measurement of the energy contained in food when digested and assimilated by the body.

cardio/aerobic Cardiovascular exercise that strengthens the heart, builds lung oxygen capacity, and releases endorphins. It needs to be sustained for a minimum of 20 minutes.

cholesterol A waxy, fatlike substance. Dietary cholesterol is found in foods of animal origin. Blood cholesterol is manufactured by the liver and found in every body cell. Cholesterol is needed for many functions of a healthy body.

complementary proteins Two or more incomplete proteins that together contain all the essential amino acids to equal a complete protein.

complete proteins Foods that contain all of the essential amino acids.

constipation The irregular, difficult, or sluggish passage of stool.

cortisol A hormone manufactured by the adrenal glands in response to stress. It facilitates fat storage and affects the immune system.

country mallow Another name used for ephedra or ma huang, the herb that is often used in thermogenic weight-loss supplements that has amphetamine-type stimulants and may have harmful side effects.

eating 0–5 Eating when you are hungry and stopping when you are satisfied, before you are full. Do this by using the hunger scale to rate the hunger and fullness of your stomach, on a scale of 0-10. Zero means that your stomach has hunger pangs and is empty. Five means that you have had enough food but not too much food. So eat from 0 up to 5. Seven means that you are full, and 10 means that you are stuffed.

eating beautifully Eating in an environment that is peaceful, health-giving, and fun.

effective weight-loss system A system that incorporates behavior, nutrition, and exercise along with education to help a person maintain his or her ideal size.

endorphins Chemical agents released by the body that stimulate the brain to feel good, released during vigorous exercise.

energy The fuel required by the body to power body processes. Energy is obtained from carbohydrate, protein, fat, and alcohol.

enzyme A protein that facilitates chemical reactions in the body.

ephedra An herb, also known as ma huang and country mallow, used in many diet supplements that has amphetamine-type stimulants and that may have harmful side effects.

essential amino acids These cannot be made by the body. They must come from food sources.

essential fatty acids   Dietary fats that the body requires for health.

fasting   The act of abstaining from eating food for a period of time, usually one or more days.

fiber   That portion of a plant that the human body cannot digest. It provides indigestible bulk, which encourages the normal elimination of body wastes.

food combining   Eating more than one kind of carbohydrate that contains incomplete proteins so that, when combined, you are consuming all the essential amino acids found in complete proteins such as meat and eggs. For instance, eating beans and rice together will provide you with all the essential amino acids. You don't have to eat the combined foods at the same meal as long as you eat them within the same 24-hour period.

forgiveness   The act of pardoning others or yourself without harboring resentment.

free radicals   Unstable, hyperactive molecules that move around in the body, damaging healthy cells and tissues.

glycemic index   A measure of a carbohydrate's ability to raise the body's blood sugar.

glycemic load   A measure of the impact a serving of carbohydrates has on a person's blood sugar levels. Glycemic load = glycemic index × grams of carbs per serving.

good nutrition   The state that exists when the body has been receiving the required amounts of the nutrients it needs to function properly.

gym   A health club, athletic center, recreation center, or other location that offers exercise facilities.

high-glycemic   A food containing rapidly digested carbohydrates, usually starches, which cause a quick rise in blood sugar and insulin levels, which can lead to increased fat storage.

hormone   A chemical substance produced by body organs that alters the functional activity of various organs in the body.

hunger   A physical sensation triggered by hormones and blood chemistry that tells you your body needs fuel.

hunger scale   A numeric system that measures hunger on a scale of 0-10. The scale is designed to help you rate the fullness of your stomach. See *eating 0–5*.

ideal size   The size that keeps you healthy and makes you happy.

incomplete proteins   Foods containing some but not all of the essential amino acids.

inertia   This law of physics states that a body in motion tends to stay in motion and a body at rest tends to stay at rest. This law applies to exercise programs and body movement in general.

insulin   A hormone secreted by the pancreas in response to rising blood sugar.

intention   A statement that is the subset of a primary affirmation.

ketosis   A body condition that occurs when the body burns fat without enough glucose.

light box   An electrical lighting device that provides natural, full-spectrum light.

liposuction   A surgical procedure in which body fat is suctioned from various fat-storage areas of the body.

long-cooking oatmeal   Steel-cut oats, usually imported from Ireland. Available at health food and specialty food stores.

ma huang   Another name for the herb ephedra that is used in thermogenic weight-loss supplements that has amphetamine-type stimulants and may have harmful side effects.

macronutrients   Nutrients required in relatively large amounts, such as calcium and phosphorus.

metabolism   The sum total of all chemical reactions that take place in living cells. Also, the rate at which a person burns calories.

micronutrients   Nutrients required in relatively small amounts, such as vanadium, which is beneficial for thyroid metabolism, and boron, which is important to bone health.

mineral   An inorganic compound occurring in nature and required by the body for normal metabolic functioning.

neurotransmitter   A chemical produced by brain cells (neurons) that increases or decreases brain activity.

nonessential amino acids   These are amino acids that can be synthesized in the body from the essential amino acids and are required for health.

nutrients   The chemical components of food that the body requires to perform the various activities associated with living.

nutrition   The relationship of food to the well-being of the body.

obesity   An excess of body fat. Guidelines: 30 percent or more over the suggested weight for height or having a BMI of 30 or higher.

overweight   An excess amount of body weight, including fat, muscle, bone, and water. Guidelines: women having more than 25 percent body fat, men having more than 20 percent; women having a waist size greater than 35 inches with a high BMI, men having a waist size greater than 40 inches with a high BMI; anyone with a BMI of 25 to 29.9.

oxidation   The process by which the tissues of the body make the energy in food available to the body.

parasympathetic nervous system   The part of the autonomic nervous system that calms the brain and body.

pedometer   A small device that counts each step taken. It is usually worn on a belt or belt loop.

phytonutrients   The chemicals in plants that protect them from harsh environmental conditions and that give them color, flavor, and aroma. These are known to aid the body in promoting the immune function and preventing diseases such as cancer and heart disease.

Pilates   A total-body conditioning approach that emphasizes both stretching and strength-training, developed by Joseph Pilates. Also known as core conditioning.

plateau   No evidence of weight loss, inches lost, or a decrease in body fat for four weeks or more.

recommended dietary allowance (RDA)   In the United States, the level of dietary intake of essential nutrients considered to be sufficient to meet the nutritional needs of most healthy individuals based on age, sex, body size, activity, and diet.

registered dietitian   A nutrition professional qualified through education and mandatory recognized professional affiliation to participate, advise, and direct in the field of nutrition.

satiety   A mechanism to tell the body that it has had enough food.

saturated fat   Fats found in most animal foods and some plants. Saturated fat is solid at room temperature.

scale   A machine that measures a person's specific gravity in relation to the earth. This measurement is called a person's weight.

scorecard   A personal exercise progress and activity record.

semolina   A hard durum wheat that's high in gluten and is used commercially in many pasta products.

serotonin   A neurotransmitter in the brain that lifts mood.

spinning   A group exercise activity offered at health clubs that uses stationary bikes. The instructor sets the pace to promote a sustained high-level cardio workout.

starvation metabolism   The slowing of the basal metabolic rate, causing the body to burn calories more slowly and build up fat stores.

strength training   A program of exercises that uses resistance to stress the muscles so that they get stronger.

stress soothers   Positive, inspiring, and uplifting alternatives to eating for stress release.

sympathetic nervous system   The part of the autonomic nervous system that moves the body into fight-or-flight mode.

synthesize   The process of manufacturing a complex substance from a simpler substance.

Tibetans   Five simple exercises that are performed 21 times each. They promote health and aid in balancing hormonal activity. When done daily, they help eliminate double chins and middle age spread.

trans-fatty acids   A type of saturated fat formed during a manufacturing process called hydrogenation, which makes the fat more shelf-stable and solid at room temperature. Current research shows that these fats cause a rise in blood cholesterol levels and are the unhealthiest types of fat.

tryptophan   An amino acid that is converted to serotonin in the brain.

unsaturated fat   Fat that is liquid at room temperature. It is found naturally in most plant oils and some animal foods.

vitamin   An organic substance required by the body in trace amounts for normal metabolic functioning.

weight-loss program   A combination of an organized eating plan, an exercise program, and behavior modifications to assist in getting to and maintaining your ideal size.

yoga   Stretching-oriented exercise that promotes balance, strength, and flexibility. It originated in India thousands of years ago.

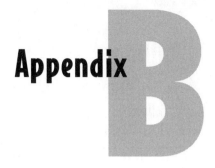

Resources

Here's where to find the products we mention as beneficial for your weight-loss and exercise success. In addition, we have given you a list of our favorite exercise videos and included the weight-loss books we discussed.

Back Roller, Also Called Ma Roller

Use for soothing stress, lightening headaches, aligning the spine, detoxing the body, and massaging acupressure points.

Body Tools
www.bodytools.com
1-800-845-6202
Fax: 415-382-8897

Be Thin in Body, Mind, & Spirit CDs

Listen to the basic concepts of weight loss as presented in this book with the *Be Thin in Body, Mind, and Spirit* CDs (2 CDs, 3 playing hours) and learn how to release spiritual and emotional toxins stored in body fat so that you can reach your ideal size.

www.LucyBeale.com
1-888-443-1979 (during business hours)

Body Rolling

Use to soothe stress, eliminate cellulite, reduce heavy musculature, and realign posture.

Body Rolling
book, video, and balls
www.yamunabodyrolling.com

FitBall® Body Therapy
book, video, and balls
www.fitball.com

Clickers and Pedometers

Use to measure the number of steps you take every day.

Available at sporting goods stores.

Exercise Videos

Use for your at-home exercise program.

www.collagevideo.com   This site has a terrific selection of tapes for Pilates, yoga, cardio, fitness ball, and more. Here you can find these instructors and videos that we recommend:

- *FitBall® Lower-Body Challenge* and *Upper-Body Challenge*. The moves on these two videos are terrific for toning, but the video is challenging. If you are just starting out, go slowly, don't get intimidated, and work up carefully to full speed.

- *Moira Stott: Pilates Matwork, Flexband and Fitness Circle Workouts*. Moira is a revered world expert in Pilates. Her deep understanding of body movement comes through in her videos.

www.FitBall.com   This site has Colleen Craig's *On The Ball* video that offers great instruction on Pilates for beginning FitBall® users.

www.stottpilates.com   This site offers all of Moira Stott's videos plus videos for using the Reformer equipment. Choose from *Essential Reformer, Intermediate Reformer, Advanced Reformer I* and *II*, and *Power Reformer* videos.

Fitness Ball

Purchase the FitBall for stretching, toning, and Pilates-type exercises.

www.fitball.com
1-800-752-2255

Fitness Circle

Purchase for Pilates-type strengthening, toning, and flexibility exercises.

www.pilates-studio.com

www.stottpilates.com

Glycemic Index

Download or print out a list of the glycemic index and load of hundreds of carbohydrates. Free.

www.mendosa.com/gi.htm

Glycemic Index and Load Software

Use this computer program to calculate the glycemic load or each serving of carbohydrates.

www.phelpsteam.com/glycoload
Costs under $20.

Internet Weight-Loss Sites

You'll find online support for losing weight and keeping it off.

www.eDiets.com

www.CyberDiets.com

www.iVillage.com

www.nutrition.about.com

Light Box

Use on cloudy or sunless days to brighten your mood, lift your spirits, and balance your hormones.

Happy Lite
Costs under $200.
www.gaiam.com

Lucy's Letter—E-mail Newsletter

Sign up to receive Lucy Beale's monthly newsletter filled with great info on weight loss, wellness, exercise, and more.

www.LucyBeale.com (to sign up)

Pilates Reformer Equipment

Purchase the ultimate Pilates workout equipment. Yes, you're worth it.

www.pilates-studio.com

www.QVC.com

www.gaiam.com

This equipment works well for home use and costs about $500.

Protein Counter

Use to plan your meals so that you eat adequate amounts of complete high-quality protein for each meal.

The Protein Counter, by Annette B. Natow, Pocket Books, March 1997.

You can also print a protein counter from the website at www.aakp.org/calorieerg.htm.

Rebounding Boots

Lift your endorphins quickly while exercising for aerobic stamina in these boots. They cushion joints with a rebounding effect. Take them with you for travel so you can easily do your daily exercise.

www.HealthMattersNow.net
1-919-967-2632

Supplements

All of these dietary supplements, unless otherwise noted, are widely available at health food stores.

- ◆ Electrolytes: Emergen-C comes in individual packets and mixes instantly with water (many different flavors). Knudsen's Recharge Drink is bottled fruit juice with electrolytes.

- ◆ Essential amino acids: Dozens of good amino acid supplements are available at health food stores. We suggest you try several to determine which brand works best for you.

- ◆ Digestive enzymes: NOW Super Enzyme Caps.

- ◆ Digestive support for protein: Country Life Betaine Hydrochloride tablets.

- ◆ Essential fatty acids (EFAs): Take 1-2 TB per day.
  Carlson's Fish Oil—Lemon Flavored. Omega 3 Fish Oil Lemon Lime by www.vitaminshoppe.com.

- ◆ Greens drinks: Great to reduce the symptoms of yeast infections. Use for stress and restoring energy as these are filled with antioxidants, too. Greens Plus at www.greensplus.com and at health food stores. Udo's Choice Wholesome Fast Food Blend.

- ◆ Liquid B vitamins: B Total Sublingual.

- ◆ Stress Support, Cortisol Lowering: Theanine in capsules at health-food stores. Corterra Xcel at www.nexagenusa.com/bethinpatch.

- ◆ Trace minerals: ConcenTrace Trace Mineral Tablets.

- ◆ Forslean: An ayurvedic herb used for centuries to release fat stores and normalize thyroid function. The primary ingredient in the Fat-Loss Patch, available at www.Lucybeale.com.

Tibetan Exercise Books

Do these exercises daily to balance hormones and eliminate double chins and midriff bulges. They make you feel great.

◆ *Ancient Secret of the Fountain of Youth, Book 1.* Peter Kelder, Bernie S. Siegel, Doubleday, February 1998. This is the original book. Reprinted from the 1939 edition.

◆ *Ancient Secret of the Fountain of Youth, Book 2.* Peter Kelder, Bernie S. Siegel, Doubleday, February 1999. This updated and expanded book explains why the exercises are so effective and includes beginner exercises for building up strength for doing the complete set of five exercises.

Weight Loss Books

◆ *The South Beach Diet*, by Arthur Agatston, M.D., Rodale, 2003.

◆ *The G.I. Diet*, by Rick Gallop, Workman, 2002.

◆ *The 3-hour Diet*, by Jorge Cruise.

◆ *The Paleo Diet*, by Loren Cordaine, Ph.D., Wiley, 2002.

◆ *The Fat Flush Plan*, by Ann Louise Gittleman, McGraw Hill, 2002.

◆ *The New Glucose Revolution*, by Jennie Brand-Miller, Thomas M. S. Wolever, Kaye Foster-Powell, Stephen Colagiura, Marlowe & Company, 1999.

◆ *Dr. Atkins New Diet Revolution*, Robert C. Atkins, M.D., Avon, December 2001.

◆ *Sugar Busters*, H. Leighton Steward; Sam S. Andrews, M.D.; Morrison C. Bethea, M.D.; Luis A. Balart, M.D.; Ballantine, May 1998.

◆ *The Zone*, Barry Sears, Ph.D., with Bill Lawren, Harper Collins, June 1995.

Yoga and Stretching

Use yoga and stretching for exercise and for soothing stress.

◆ *Bikram's Beginning Yoga Class*, Bikram Choudhury, J. P. Tarcher, August 2000.

◆ *Stretching*, Bob Anderson, Shelter, 2002.

Index

X-Y-Z

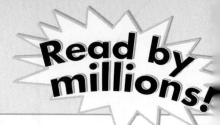
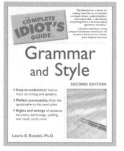
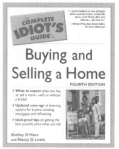
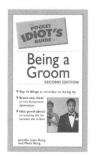
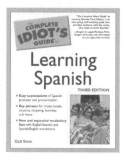
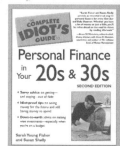
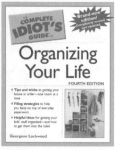
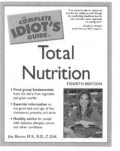
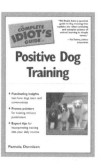
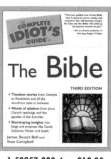
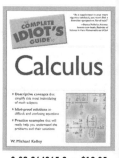
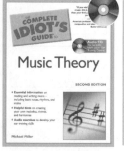
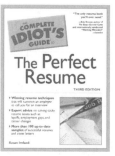
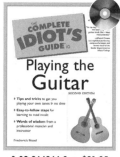
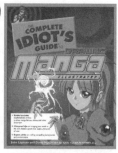
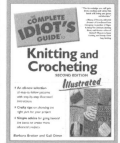